Women and Well-Being
Les femmes et le mieux-être

WOMEN AND WELL-BEING
LES FEMMES ET LE MIEUX-ÊTRE

**EDITED BY/SOUS LA DIRECTION DE
VANAJA DHRUVARAJAN**

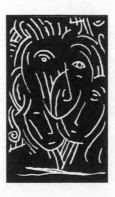

Published for/publié pour
The Canadian Research Institute for the Advancement of Women
l'Institut canadien de recherches sur les femmes

by/par
McGill–Queen's University Press
Montreal & Kingston • London • Buffalo

Legal deposit third quarter 1990
Bibliothèque nationale du Québec

Printed in Canada on acid-free paper

Canadian Cataloguing in Publication Data

Main entry under title:
Women and well-being =
Les femmes et le mieux-être
Text in English and French.
ISBN 0-7735-0734-5 (bound). –
ISBN 0-7735-0762-0 (pbk.)
1. Women – Health and hygiene – Canada –
Sociological aspects. 2. Women – Mental health –
Canada – Sociological aspects. 3. Women – Canada
– Social conditions. I. Dhruvarajan, Vanaja II.
Canadian Research Institute for the Advancement
of Women III. Title: Les Femmes et le mieux-être.
HQ1106.W653 1990   362.1'082   C90-090341-4E

Données de catalogage avant publication (Canada)

Vedette principale au titre:
Women and well-being =
Les femmes et le mieux-être
Textes en anglais et en français.
ISBN 0-7735-0734-5 (relié). –
ISBN 0-7735-0762-0 (br.)
1. Femmes – Santé et hygiène – Canada – Aspect
sociologique. 2. Femmes – Santé mentale – Canada
– Aspect sociologique. 3. Femmes – Canada –
Conditions sociales. I. Dhruvarajan, Vanaja II.
Institut canadien de recherches sur les femmes III.
Titre: Les Femmes et le mieux-être.
HQ1106.W653 1990   362.1'082   C90-090341-4F

This book was typeset by
Typo Litho composition inc.
in 10/12 Baskerville.

Contents
Table des Matières

WOMEN, KNOWLEDGE, AND WELL-BEING/LES FEMMES, LA CONNAISSANCE, ET LE MIEUX-ÊTRE

Acknowledgments
Remerciements

Publication of this collection of articles has been made possible through the efforts of many. Here I thank only those who have contributed directly: the 1987 CRIAW Conference organizing committee – Gail Hall, Melba Crookshanks, Katherine Schultz, Mavis Turner, co-chaired by myself and Hilary Lips – for their planning, dedication, and hard work; Diane McGifford and Judy Kearns for proofreading the articles in English and Diane for helping me edit several articles; Monique Raimbault for summarizing the French articles and proofreading them; Linda O'Neil for providing help whenever I needed it, which I did quite often; Peta Tancred-Sheriff for sharing her valuable insights into the job of editing; Judi Hanson and Bea Wong for efficiently word processing the collection; the University of Winnipeg for the help provided by various staff members; the Canadian Research Institute for the Advancement of Women and the Women's Program, Secretary of State, for their financial assistance towards the publication of this volume; and finally all the authors who took pains in writing these articles.

Les efforts de nombreuses personnes ont rendu possible la publication de ce recueil d'articles. Je ne peux remercier ici que celles qui ont apporté une contribution directe : Gail Hall, Melba Crookshanks, Katherine Schultz et Mavis Turner, membres du comité organisateur du colloque de l'ICREF de 1987 – dont j'ai assumé la présidence conjointement avec Hilary Lips – pour leur planification, leur dévouement et leur travail acharné; Diane McGifford et Judy Kearns, qui ont corrigé ensemble les épreuves des articles anglais – Diane m'a également aidée à mettre au point plusieurs articles; Monique Raimbault, qui a résumé les articles français et en a corrigé les épreuves; Linda O'Neil, qui m'a apporté son aide chaque fois que j'en ai eu besoin – ce qui s'est produit souvent; Peta Tancred-Sheriff, qui m'a fait profiter de sa connaissance de l'édition; Judi Hanson et Bea Wong, qui ont assuré le traitement de texte avec efficacité; l'Université de Winnipeg, pour l'aide que m'ont apportée divers membres de son personnel; l'Institut canadien de recherches sur les femmes et le Programme de la promotion de la femme du Secrétariat d'État pour leur contribution financière à la publication de ce volume; et enfin toutes les auteures qui se sont donné la peine de rédiger ces articles.

Preface
Préface

This collection of twenty articles is selected from the 1987 CRIAW conference proceedings. Before these articles are introduced, I would like to mention some of the highlights of the conference. The conference, held in Winnipeg from 6 to 8 November, was attended by close to 350 people and provided an intellectually stimulating and emotionally exhilarating experience. As always with CRIAW conferences, the conference expressed feminist visions for a better world and a deep yearning for its realization.

The most significant event was the plenary session, which was attended by all the holders of federally funded chairs in Women's Studies, past and present, except for the holder of the chair at Laval, since that appointment had not been made. Each participant elaborated on the issues most dear to her, revealing her own unique professional and personal experiences. Monique Bégin, at the University of Ottawa and Carleton University, and Rosemary Brown, at Simon Fraser University, have extensive experience in the political sphere. Marguerite Andersen at Mount Saint Vincent University and Keith Louise Fulton at University of Manitoba and University of Winnipeg are respectively scholars of French and English literature. Susan Penfold at Simon Fraser University (past chair) is a psychiatrist and Thelma McCormack at Mount Saint Vincent (past chair) is a sociologist. The session gave a glimpse into what is involved in being a chairperson, what has been accomplished and what remains to be accomplished, and, of course, what joys and sorrows are involved in the endeavour.

One of the most inspiring moments of the conference was the introduction of Jerilynn Celia Prior, the recipient of the Muriel Duckworth Award. A peaceactivist and a feminist, Jerilynn has dedicated her life to promoting the well-being of all people. It was indeed a privilege to get to know this remarkable person.

There was the thought-provoking opening address by Monique
Bégin, which appears here, and close to fifty papers and workshops
from which the articles included in this volume were chosen. Hu-
mourous and thoughtful entertainment was provided by Manitoba's
own Nellie McClung Theatre, Contemporary Dancers, Heidi
Hunter, Suzanne Campagne, and Tracy Riley. All of this made me
feel – in spite of the trials and tribulations that go with organizing
a conference – glad to have been a part of it.

Les vingt articles qui suivent sont tirés des actes du colloque de 1987
de l'ICREF. Avant de les présenter, j'aimerais souligner quelques faits
saillants de ce colloque tenu à Winnipeg du 6 au 8 novembre 1987.
Près de 350 personnes ont participé à cette expérience intellectuelle
et émotive, stimulante et vivifiante. Comme à l'habitude, le colloque
s'est déroulé dans une atmosphère de visions féministes d'un monde
meilleur animées d'un vif désir d'en voir la concrétisation.

L'événement marquant fut la séance plénière qui réunissait
notamment toutes les titulaires passées et actuelles des chaires d'études sur la condition des femmes, subventionnées par le gouvernement fédéral, à l'exception de la titulaire de la chaire de l'Université
Laval qui n'avait pas encore été nommée. Chacune a traité des questions qui lui tenaient le plus à coeur en faisant le récit de ses expériences professionnelles et personnelles. Monique Bégin, des
Universités d'Ottawa et Carleton, et Rosemary Brown, de l'Université
Simon Fraser, jouissent d'une vaste expérience du monde politique;
Marguerite Andersen, de l'Université Mount Saint Vincent, et Keith
Louise Fulton, des Universités du Manitoba et de Winnipeg, sont
spécialistes en littérature française et anglaise respectivement; Susan
Penfold, ancienne titulaire à l'Université Simon Fraser, est psychiatre, et Thelma McCormack, ancienne titulaire à l'Université Mount
Saint Vincent, est sociologue. La séance a donné un aperçu du poste
de titulaire de chaire, du chemin parcouru et à parcourir et, évi-
demment, des joies et des peines inhérentes aux fonctions de ce
poste.

L'un des moments les plus émouvants du colloque fut la présentation de Jerilynn Celia Prior, récipiendaire du prix Muriel
Duckworth. Pacifiste et féministe, Jerilynn a consacré sa vie à la
promotion du mieux-être de toutes et tous. Ce fut un réel privilège
de mieux connaître cette personne remarquable.

Monique Bégin a prononcé une allocution d'ouverture qui a sti-
mulé la réflexion et que nous reproduisons dans ce volume. Il y eut
également près de cinquante communications et ateliers dont sont

extraits les articles qui suivent. Le Manitoba a fourni les divertisse-
ments à la fois humoristiques et bien pensés, qui ont étés offerts par
des troupes du Manitoba dont le Nellie McClung Theatre, les Contemporary Dancers de Heidi Hunter, Suzanne Campagne et Tracy
Riley. Bref, tout a contribué à ma satisfaction de pouvoir participer
à ce colloque, malgré les soucis et les tribulations qui accompagnent
inévitablement l'organisation d'un tel événement.

Introduction

The common theme in this collection is concern about women's well-being. In the chapters that follow, this concern is expressed by identifying conditions that are congenial or detrimental to women's well-being and by exploring ways and means of promoting it. The authors come from a variety of backgrounds and state the issues from their own vantage points choosing topics that interest them and adopting different theoretical and disciplinary frameworks.

The twenty chapters in this collection are divided into four parts on the basis of the particular aspects of women's well-being they address. The five chapters in Part I deal with issues concerning women's physical and mental health and well-being. In the first chapter, Monique Bégin, drawing upon her extensive experience in the Canadian political arena, critically evaluates the biomedical model adopted by the Canadian health care system and points out how it fails to effectively promote women's well-being. She suggests alternative models and highlights the need for political discussion of issues from the private arena. In the second chapter, basing her observations on the analyses of three novels, Andrea Lebowitz shows how women writers have used women's bodily health and illness to explain women's status and make statements about their well-being in a patriarchal socio-cultural context. In addition to the cultural imagery of women's bodies and women's felt need to gain approval from men, Dawn Currie, in chapter 3, draws our attention to the material conditions of women's lives that lead to the development of anorexia and bulimia, which threaten women's health and well-being. The next chapter, by Doris McIlroy, highlights the fact that social class differences among women are real and must be taken into account in explaining the kinds of body images women develop, which can have implications for their well-being. Megan Barker

Davies, in the last chapter of this part, concerns herself with the well-being of women in mental health institutions in the early part of this century. She shows how gender stereotyping was reinforced in these institutions and how women followed gender-specific strategies in coping with the stresses of institutional life.

The five chapters in Part 2 deal with issues of concern for women's well-being in the area of work in both the private and public spheres. The first chapter in this part draws attention to the fact that the well-being of the caregivers, as well as that of the care recipients, should be an issue. Nancy Guberman critically evaluates the position taken by government agencies, families, and society in general, showing that the well-being of caregivers (who are almost always women) is completely ignored. Leslie Bella analyses the threats to the well-being of women when the conception of leisure is androcentric. Taking the example of Christmas, she shows how women's labour produces family leisure. She elaborates on society's prevalent conviction that women should be in charge of such labour. Caroline Andrew, Cécile Coderre, and Ann Denis discuss the issue of integrating family and career life to insure women's sense of well-being. Based on a study that delineates the work and family environments of women in management, the authors argue that integration of career and family life has been possible for these women and they are happier for it. Ghyslaine Savaria points out that women involved in family businesses are at risk because of the lack of legal recognition of their business partnerships with their husbands. Documenting the role played by the women's association that she represents, she stresses the importance of such associations in raising women's awareness of the need to protect their own economic well-being. Gloria Geller discusses the kinds of threats that women who venture into nontraditional jobs experience to their well-being. Drawing upon her study of ten women working in correctional institutions, Geller shows how women bring unique talents and experiences to the situation and how they try to transcend the difficulties they face.

Part 3 discusses the relationship between well-being and minority status. Each author elaborates on the consequences of such status for a particular group of women. In the first chapter, Eva Szeleky shows that it is necessary to take into account both the class and racial background of immigrants in order to assess their sense of well-being. She identifies the kinds of dangers involved for these women's well-being if only class differences are addressed and racial and ethnic differences are relegated to the cultural arena. Kabahenda Nyakabwa and Carol Harvey identify the challenges and threats to their sense of well-being that black immigrant women face.

These include all the problems faced by other immigrant women in addition to prejudice and discrimination because of their historical legacy of slavery and colonization. Monique Raimbault shows how the well-being of women with disabilities is threatened because of their double jeopardy – being women and disabled. Based on their perceptions about their own conditions, she delineates the vulnerabilities of women with disabilities and suggests possible solutions. Based on a study of never-married elderly women's perceptions and evaluations of their own life, Mary O'Brien questions the negative stereotypes prevalent in the literature regarding the lives of elderly women. She argues that the women in her sample experience a sense of well-being and a feeling of life well lived. Madeline Graveline points out how rural women, because they are isolated from the larger society and more restricted by patriarchal culture, experience a low sense of well-being. She highlights the need for the women's movement to reach these women to let them build better lives for themselves.

Authors of the five chapters in Part 4 concern themselves with ensuring the well-being of women by empowering them through knowledge. In the first chapter in this part, Claire de la Durantaye argues that women's ways of knowing, being, and doing, which emphasize harmony, connection, and completeness, are qualitatively different from those of men, who are obsessed with objectivity and control. She argues that men's perspectives are essentially dehumanizing and therefore women's perspectives should be promoted to ensure the well-being of humanity. In the next chapter, taking the example of mature women who had not gone through the school system in their younger days, Elayne Harris speaks to the conviction that knowledge gained through reading and writing enhances self-esteem and the sense of well-being. She shows that this objective is best accomplished by providing opportunities for women to learn as they are doing something meaningful for themselves and their communities. Joanne Prindiville and Cathryn Boak discuss the issue of the empowerment of women in the community through long-distance delivery of courses in Women's Studies. They point out the need for caution, since such knowledge can pose a threat to the well-being of those women situated in patriarchal families. Maureen Leyland and Maureen Jessop Orton, drawing on their research, argue strongly in favour of educating adolescents about reproductive functions in order to prevent teenage pregnancy. They show how it is detrimental to the interests of adolescents, especially those in lower socioeconomic classes, if those in positions of power maintain a moralistic stance and exercise control over the dissemination of

this information. In the last chapter, Marguerite Andersen argues
that the theme of love, which engulfs the lives of women in so many
ways, has been a source of danger and despair that affects women's
well-being. She expresses the hope that growing awareness among
women through the betterment of their status will lead to love as a
source of life rather than a destructive force.

Since this collection consists of many thoughtful insights into the
issue of well-being, it makes for fascinating reading. But, more importantly, it has the potential not only to inform but also to empower
women.

Les textes de ce recueil traitent d'une préoccupation commune, le
mieux-être des femmes. Cette préoccupation se manifeste dans la
définition de conditions qui favorisent le mieux-être ou lui nuisent
et dans la recherche de moyens pour y parvenir. Les auteures aux
antécédents variés énoncent les problèmes à partir de leur situation
particulière, choisissant les sujets qui les touchent et adoptant des
cadres théoriques ou disciplinaires différents.

Les vingt articles de ce recueil se répartissent en quatre sections,
selon les aspects particuliers du mieux-être des femmes dont ils traitent. Les cinq articles de la première section examinent les questions
de santé et de bien-être d'ordre physique et mental. Dans le premier,
Monique Bégin puise dans sa vaste expérience de l'arène politique
canadienne pour faire une évaluation critique du modèle biomédical
adopté par le système canadien de services de santé et signale à quel
point ce modèle ne réussit pas à améliorer la condition des femmes.
Elle propose des substituts et insiste sur la nécessité d'un débat politique sur des questions du domaine privé. Dans le deuxième article,
Andrea Lebowitz, s'inspirant d'une analyse de trois romans, montre
comment les écrivaines ont invoqué l'état physique des femmes pour
parler de leur condition et de leur mieux-être dans un contexte socio-
culturel patriarcal. En plus de nous décrire l'image du corps féminin
inhérente à notre culture et cette obligation que ressentent les femmes d'avoir l'approbation des hommes, Dawn Currie attire notre
attention dans le troisième article, sur la situation matérielle des
femmes qui les conduit à l'anorexie et à la boulimie et menace leur
santé et leur bien-être. Dans l'article suivant, Doris McIlroy nous fait
remarquer que les différentes classes sociales des femmes sont une
réalité et soutient qu'il faut en tenir compte pour expliquer l'image
que se font les femmes de leur corps et qui peut avoir des répercussions sur leur mieux-être. Dans le dernier article de cette section,
Megan Barker Davies se penche sur le mieux-être des femmes dans

les établissements de santé mentale au début du siècle. Elle nous fait voir comment ces établissements favorisaient les stéréotypes sexistes et nous indique les stratégies que les femmes ont adoptées pour surmonter le stress engendré par la vie en établissement.

Les cinq articles de la deuxième section traitent de préoccupations relatives au mieux-être professionnel des femmes dans les secteurs public et privé. La premier attire l'attention sur la nécessité de tenir compte du mieux-être tant des personnes qui prodiguent des soins que de celles qui les reçoivent. Nancy Guberman fait une évaluation critique de la position adoptée par les organismes gouvernementaux, les familles et la société en général qui laissent complètement pour compte le mieux-être des personnes qui donnent les soins, presque toujours des femmes. Leslie Bella étudie en détail les embûches pour le mieux-être des femmes qu'entraîne une conception androcentrique des loisirs. Prenant Noël comme exemple, elle montre comment les loisirs familiaux dépendent du travail des femmes. Elle s'étend sur les convictions généralisées d'une société qui estime que ce sont les femmes qui doivent assumer cette tâche. Caroline Andrew, Cécile Coderre et Ann Denis examinent la façon dont une femme peut concilier famille et profession et se sentir bien. En se basant sur une étude qui décrit le milieu familial et le milieu de travail de femmes gestionnaires, les auteures soutiennent que ces femmes ont réussi à concilier les deux, ce qui leur a permis d'être plus heureuses. Ghyslaine Savaria signale à quel point les femmes oeuvrant dans des entreprises familiales courent des risques en raison du manque de reconnaissance juridique de leur partenariat avec leur conjoint. Expliquant le rôle de l'association de femmes qu'elle représente, l'auteure insiste sur l'importance de ces associations qui sensibilisent les femmes à la nécessité de protéger leur mieux-être économique. Gloria Geller discute des risques que prennent les femmes qui s'aventurent dans des emplois non traditionnels. Elle se reporte à l'étude qu'elle a réalisée avec dix femmes employées dans des établissements correctionnels pour montrer comment les femmes font intervenir leurs expériences et leurs talents particuliers dans leur travail et essaient de surmonter les difficultés auxquelles elles se heurtent.

Chacun des articles de la troisième partie établit le rapport entre le mieux-être et la situation des minorités. Chaque auteure s'attarde aux conséquences de cette situation pour un groupe de femmes particulier. Le premier article, signé par Eva Szekely, démontre la nécessité de tenir compte tant de la classe sociale que de la race des immigrantes pour bien évaluer leur sentiment de mieux-être. Selon l'auteure, le fait de ne tenir compte que des différences sociales de ces femmes et de reléguer les différences raciales ou ethniques au domaine culturel compromet ce bien-être. Kabahenda Nyakabwa et Carol Harvey traitent des problèmes des immigrantes noires, c'est-à-dire de tous ceux auxquels se heurtent les autres immigrantes en plus des préjugés et de la discrimination hérités de leur longue histoire d'esclavage et de colonisation. Dans l'article suivant, Monique Raimbault montre comment le mieux-être des femmes handicapées est compromis par une double réalité : être femme et être handicapée. S'inspirant des perceptions mêmes de ces femmes, elle décrit leurs points vulnérables et propose des solutions. Mary O'Brien, pour sa part, fait appel à une étude sur la perception qu'ont les femmes âgées célibataires de leur vie et conteste les stéréotypes que l'on retrouve à l'égard de ces femmes dans la littérature. Elle soutient que les femmes qui ont participé à son expérience éprouvent un sentiment de mieux-être et de vie bien remplie. Madeline Jean Graveline nous montre à quel point les femmes en milieu rural se réjouissent peu de leur état à cause de leur isolement et des contraintes plus rigoureuses de la culture patriarcale. Elle signale la nécessité pour le mouvement féministe de rejoindre ces femmes pour leur permettre de se bâtir une meilleure vie.

Les auteures des cinq articles de la quatrième partie relient le mieux-être des femmes à l'acquisition du pouvoir par le biais du savoir. Dans le premier article, Claire de la Durantaye soutient que la manière de connaître, d'être et d'agir des femmes, qui s'articule autour de l'harmonie, des relations et de la plénitude, est qualitativement différente de celle des hommes, qui sont obsédés par l'objectivité et la domination. Elle ajoute que les perspectives masculines sont essentiellement déshumanisantes et que, par conséquent, il faut promouvoir les perspectives féminines pour assurer le mieux-être de l'humanité. Dans l'article suivant, Elaine Harris prend l'exemple de femmes d'âge mûr qui n'ont pas fréquenté l'école dans leur enfance et se dit convaincue que la connaissance acquise par la lecture et l'écriture favorise l'estime de soi et le sentiment de mieux-être. Elle nous montre que le meilleur moyen d'atteindre cet objectif est de donner aux femmes l'occasion d'apprendre tout en faisant quelque chose de significatif pour elles-mêmes et pour leur collectivité. Joanne Prindiville et Cathryn Boak se penchent sur l'enseignement à distance de cours d'études sur les femmes, et sur le pouvoir que les femmes dans les collectivités peuvent ainsi acquérir. Elles préviennent cependant que la prudence est nécessaire, car ces connaissances peuvent constituer une menace au mieux-être des femmes en milieu patriarcal. Les recherches de Maureen Leyland et de Maureen Jessop Orten leur permettent de soutenir vigoureusement que les adolescentes doivent mieux connaître les fonctions du système de reproduction si elles veulent un meilleur contrôle de leur vie. Les auteures font valoir à quel point le maintien d'une attitude moraliste et la restriction de la diffusion de cette information par les personnes au pouvoir peuvent être préjudiciables aux intérêts des adolescentes, particulièrement celles des classes inférieures. Dans le dernier article, Marguerite Andersen soutient que le thème de l'amour dans lequel s'engouffrent les femmes à tant d'égards a été une source de danger et de désespoir. Elle exprime l'espoir que la sensibilisation croissante des femmes grâce à l'amélioration de leur condition les mènera à l'amour source de vie plutôt que force destructive.

La lecture de ce recueil est captivante, grâce aux observations sérieuses qu'il réunit sur le mieux-être des femmes. Mais ce qui est encore plus important, c'est qu'en plus d'être une source de renseignements, il offre aux femmes la possibilité de s'approprier plus de pouvoir.

Women, Health, and Well-Being
Les femmes, la santé, et le mieux-être

MONIQUE BÉGIN

Redesigning Health Care for Women[1]

Monique Bégin addresses the issue of women and health. Women and
the elderly have been badly served by modern medicine because reproduction and the aging process are not pathological states but are changes
in health status and for this reason do not interest medical research.
Bégin looks at the excessive power of physicians and other experts; at the
internal logic of the biomedical model of health; and at the profound
ambivalence of health-care users and the public in general toward the
miracles of science and technology. What do women want in health care?
Bégin examines demedicalization, changes in attitudes, alternative practices, and collaboration with women health-care professionals. Her conclusion denounces the social contradictions in the roles imposed on
women and the price that women pay in health, both physical and
mental.

Nouveau concept des soins de santé pour les femmes

Ce texte se veut un essai sur la problématique « femmes et santé. » Il
pose d'abord le constat que les femmes (et les personnes âgées) ont été
mal servies par la médecine moderne puisque la fonction de reproduction
chez les femmes et le vieillissement chez les gens âgés ne sont pas des
maladies mais bien des variations dans l'état de santé. À ce titre, ni l'un ni
l'autre n'intéressent la recherche médicale. La réflexion se porte ensuite
sur le pouvoir excessif des médecins et autres experts et expertes, la
logique interne du modèle biomédical et la profonde ambivalence des
usagères et usagers et du public en général envers les miracles de la
science et de la technologie. Suit une analyse de ce que veulent les femmes: démédicalisation, changement d'attitudes, pratiques alternatives, collaboration avec les professionnel-le-s de la santé. L'essai se termine sur
une dénonciation des contradictions sociales dans les rôles imposés aux

femmes et du prix qu'elles en payent dans leur santé physique et mentale.

Recently, someone reminded me that the Report of the Royal Commission on the Status of Women in Canada did not address the issue of women and health. Indeed, when I recall the hundreds of briefs, the numerous public hearings, and the final report and recommendations tabled in December 1970, which I co-signed with the commissioners, I cannot remember that anyone dealt with this issue.[2] Yet almost seventeen years later, this entire CRIAW conference is devoted to the theme of "Women and Well-being." As well, I myself am teaching courses on women and health in two universities. In October 1987, I attended the International Forum on New Reproductive Technologies organized jointly by the Advisory Council on the Status of Women of the Quebec government and by the Simone de Beauvoir Institute of Concordia University, in Montreal.[3] The conference organizers received 1,050 applications to attend and had to refuse 500 due to lack of space.

Given the current interest in women's health care, the silence of the Royal Commission Report is puzzling. An explanation for that silence can, however, be found. When Lester B. Pearson established the Royal Commission on the Status of Women in the late 1960s, women were working to achieve simple justice in their daily lives. They sought equal pay for equal work ("work of equal value" would come later), the use of their own names, access to independent lines of credit in business transactions, parental rather than paternal family responsibility, equal access to assets acquired by the couple after marriage, training courses to enable re-entry into the paid labour force after raising children, and so on. The list of urgently required simple justice issues was long.

During the same period (1967–70), great national excitement greeted the implementation of the Medical Care Act – our "Medicare." This program did not lead to doubts or questions. Rather, all segments of our society worshipped the biomedical model of health care and its many breakthroughs. In those years, Candians sought more access to more medical care. While the Boston Women's Health Care Collective began addressing malpractice in 1969 – research that culminated in the first edition of the now famous *Our Bodies, Ourselves* (1971) – the consumer's movement in general had yet to question the standard medical practice. Only very slowly and somewhat tardily did the Canadian public begin to question the authoritarian mode of interaction between medical care providers and patients, the overspecialization and extreme fragmentation of the health-care system, and, above all, the ever increasing medicalization of life. Although the popularity of alternative medicines (that is, those health procedures not covered by our provincial health plans), on which Canadians spend millions of dollars, testifies to the limits of the conventional biomedical model, audiences are still very surprised – almost aggressively so – when they are confronted with evidence that, beyond a certain point of accessibility, more medical care cannot increase the general health of the population.

Although many of us have been badly served by a health care system that too often believes that medicine is a science and forgets that it is, above all, an art – the art of healing – I would submit that those who have been mistreated the most have been women and the elderly. These groups suffer not only from various diseases but also from malaises and problems of body readjustment which medicine, until very recently, has not considered to be interesting. While the elderly experience health problems because of the aging process, throughout their lives women meet many problems associated with reproductive functions. Such problems have been reduced to diseases, badly diagnosed, and too often badly treated. This process alienates the patients and weakens those women who have consulted the medical care system and have consequently been divested of their own inner resources.

Prevention and health promotion are still the poor relatives of the health care system; nevertheless, our environment must be considered an important aspect of our health. The term "environment" includes such concrete factors as the level of noise or radiation emitted by one's work equipment, poverty, and malnutrition, as well as less easily defined factors derived from the psychosocial conditions of one's roles in society, such as social pressure, stress due to contradictory expectations, lack of support in family and domestic life, dependency, and lack of status. Good health goes beyond a strictly medical definition and is best expressed by the concept of well-being – the very theme of this conference. And we, as participants, will look at issues ranging from "Creating Support Networks" to "Shiatsu," from "Farm Women in Economic Crisis" to "The Case of Depo-Provera" to "Human Genetics." Neither life nor health should be divided into discrete territories, and women, perhaps more than men, are holistic in their approaches and possess a strong sense of the whole person.

Given these preliminary remarks, we must ask a few questions. Do Canadian women in large numbers discuss their needs in relation to our health care system? Are the issues of women and health on the political agenda, federally and provincially? Does each women's association have Women and Health as one of the points of its annual program, with the relevant subcommittees, studies, discussions, briefs, and resolutions? Are Women and Health courses taught in all faculties of medicine and in all schools of nursing? The list of questions could go on. In my opinion the answer, unfortunately, is no to every one of them. This is the state of affairs despite the energetic work of the Canadian women's health movement and the excellent work of *Healthsharing* magazine, despite the women's health clinics and the important role of Inter-Pares and Women's Health Interaction, and despite the *Essai sur la santé des femmes*, that remarkable book prepared by women and published by the Québec government. If we can speak of a common knowledge and experience of the issues of women and health in Canada today, we owe it entirely to these initiatives and to the networking of the women's movement. And even if, here and there, committed and genuinely caring individuals do teach courses dealing with women and health in schools of nursing and in other disciplines, the daily practice of health care in Canada still does not deal justly with women.

What then, are the objectives we should pursue at this time?

It seems to me that we should first explore the goal of the demedicalization of life. Three quite distinct approaches coexist under the heading of demedicalization. The first of these I will refer to as the radical approach. The radical approach involves choices ranging from a rejection of traditional Western medicine in favour of alternative, soft medicines, to self-examination and the development of self-help groups by women. The second approach may be referred to as the moderate approach and seeks less medicalization of life. The moderate approach incorporates such initiatives as the agenda of the Canadian Institute of Child Health for humanizing childbirth procedures and policies. The third approach to the demedicalization of life I would call the demystification of health care and therapy. By demanding information and by exploring the way the system works, patients and general consumers will be able to make informed choices within a demystified health care system.

Why does demedicalization suggest so many different meanings? To further our understanding we must question and examine the values that we privilege in our society. When it comes to actual health care delivery, no matter how radical one may wish to be, one must ask what choices one would make after learning of a diagnosis of (say) breast cancer or heart defect. Often the answer would be: "The best treatment, immediately" – that is, the most scientifically advanced treatment. Why are a large number of people choosing either the most sophisticated treatment offered by the biomedical model or, paradoxically, supplementing these procedures with alternative approaches to healing? Here lies the key to any possible change in the health care system: the strength of the biomedical model is founded upon our seemingly absolute faith in science and technology.

It is pointless, therefore, to look around for a convenient scapegoat. Although physicians and medical experts are natural targets for women's anger, the exaggerated political power such professionals enjoy in our society is conferred by us. We empower them. Our blind faith in science and technology is the cornerstone of our value system. This faith represents our vision of progress in this second half of the twentieth century. We must learn to question these fundamental beliefs and consequently the ideology which has legitimized the immense power we have given to specialist physicians as experts. Our actions will be all the more revolutionary and significant if they are solidly rooted in a thorough consideration of the relevant underlying values. This process concerns each of us in our own personal beliefs and it is a demanding experience. To what extent are we familiar with the limitations of science? What do we know of its economics, its priorities, its internal logic? To what extent have we erased from our consciences the meaning of suffering, aging, and dying – that is, the meaning of vulnerability? What have we learned from the critique made by Ivan Illich (Illich 1976) and how much acceptance has his thesis gained?

I believe that many people, myself included, react in an ambivalent manner when confronted with these questions. To this day, I am incapable of reconciling the following contradiction: How can we accept only the positive elements and reject the negative elements of modern science when the internal logic of biomedical research insists that all things must be explored in an eclectic fashion and in total freedom, and when the internal logic of the health care system is to use to the utmost the practical applications and the technology of biomedical research? I fully understand intellectually Illich's thesis that it is necessary, as a first step in dealing with iatrogenic (physician-induced) disease, to investigate global inefficiency and the dangers of our expensive health care systems. But when I was Minister of National Health, I increased the budgets of medical research programs and protected existing provincial health-care budgets while at the same time deliberately refusing to ask Cabinet to increase the budgets of the latter – despite the requests of my officials. In other words, I was unable to translate my intellectual understanding into political action. A part of me would not cooperate. And that part corresponds to the thousands of women, children, and men who live in hope of being saved by medicine and by science.

Faced with an inability to solve on a theoretical basis this contradiction, I believe that the best safeguard and the greatest wisdom is to judge each case on its own merits, to adopt a pragmatic approach, and above all to return constantly to the fundamental questions. Slowly, as if we were blind, we must clear the road and locate new landmarks. For me the work of Louise Hanvey and Shirley Post at the Canadian Institute for Child Health (CICH), represents an appropriate model for this endeavour.

In 1980, the CICH surveyed 567 hospitals to assess their maternity care and then reassessed them in 1985 to determine if there had been a decrease in dependency upon obstetrical technology, a humanizing of the care of mothers and fewer unnecessary or risky routine hospital practices and procedures (for example, perineal shaves, enemas or suppositories, intravenous therapy, electronic fetal heart monitoring, episiotomies, and so on). As they hoped, they did discover some progress – small steps towards the demedicalization of maternity care. Such research and action programs, as well as the work done by many in Ontario on midwifery, gives women the information and the tools necessary to fight the system and to make their own choices. Such approaches are clearly focused. They have the potential to affect a great number of women, both as users and providers of health care.

The Ontario Task Force Report on Midwifery, led by Mary Eberts, has recently been released. Here is another example of possible demedicalization of a life event – giving birth. Now we must wait to see what the provincial government will do with it. One thing is certain: the fact that the provincial health minister, Elinor Caplan, is a woman does not mean that the report will be implemented more quickly or more easily. As a politician, Caplan must work with the internal logic of politics and government. And you may also be certain that organized medicine and (to a degree) organized nursing will do everything possible to oppose or to control any official recognition of midwives. I have read the report summary and recommendations and there are parts of it that I am not quite certain about. In particular, I am unsure of the exact place of midwives in the health care structure and the nature of their training. But if the goal is to offer alternativies and to broaden the choices of future mothers, the principal issue is to ensure that the official recognition of midwives offers real alternatives, including both a demedicalization of pregnancy and the possibility of home births.

Earlier I mentioned how important the Canadian Institute of Child Health report was in passing on information to women. This brings me to the second objective of Women and Health research and action: the empowerment of women, as users of the health care system. How can women achieve better health care if they feel powerless and alienated in the face of established medical institutions? Empowerment is restoring to the individual woman her dignity and sense of purpose. Empowerment is also getting rid of the myths, prejudices, and preconceived notions about ourselves and our bodies, notions which are often more damaging than we perceive. Surely an important dimension of empowering women in terms of health care is the acknowledgement (if nothing else) of the incredible contradictions within the new roles women are expected to perform and the consequent effects of stress, overwork, and poor resources and status.

Empowering women to discuss their health, to control it, and to make decisions about it is, therefore, our second objective. For feminists, the first goal within this broad objective has been the reappropriation of the body. That is, women must cease to be the objects of (male) scientific investigation and instead become subjects responsible for their own bodies and health. Many factors linked to contemporary western civilization – from our lifestyles to our value systems – are responsible for the fact that all of us, women and men, have lost a sense of our bodies even though we seem to be liberated both in dress and sexual behaviour. We do not know our bodies very well; they are strangers to us. We believe that everything can be reduced to good organization, and that with this, all crises can be controlled. In the same manner, the mechanistic view of the body conveyed by medicine also defines the body as an object – something apart from the self. Surely trying to make ourselves to fit the stereotype – the 32.5-year-old urban profesional woman who manages a career, a relationship, and two perfect children – will not help us to rediscover our bodies!

The empowerment of women, besides involving consciousness-raising and a reappropriation of the body, involves the passing on of information so that all of us will be able to be equal partners in the patient-doctor relationship. As a user of the health care system, I am convinced that the many problems women face in the health care system are a result of the tendency of medical science to reduce women to their reproductive function. This is seen as their only medically interesting dimension. Menopause, for example, is only interesting when it is pathological.

This reduction of women to reproductive machines is compounded by the model followed by scientific medicine: "In its most simple formation ... [the biomedical model] maintains that each cell in the body functions solely on the basis of its genetic instructions and that external influences have little effect on the behaviour of the cell, except insofar as they can alter or mutate genetic information or penetrate the cell [membrane] and do damage to the cell." (Berliner 1984). In other words, the body consists of a number of independent (though interconnected) elements and each may be studied separately. Consequently, any organ or part of the body can be examined, repaired, modified, removed, or replaced without affecting the rest of the body. And, of course, the somatic functions of the body remain independent of the mind. In this way, women, reduced to reproductive machinery, are stripped of their strength as whole persons.

Another problem the health-care system poses for women is that it is a microcosm of society. Patriarchy, capitalism (in the US), sexism: every disease of society is also found in our medical care system. Medicine is practised within an extremely authoritarian, hierarchical, impersonal, and distant organization. In addition, modern medicine is overspecialized and hence very fragmented in its application and is most alienating for the patient. The structure of power is a vertical one with the (male) physician at the top, the (female) nurse as an obedient and respectful assistant, and the patient as a passive creature, an infant, at the bottom. We may assume that this mode of relationship is even more damaging for women than for men since our socialization and the prevalent ideologies and power structures favour the conventional hierarchy and reinforce the traditional model of medical care. Learning of the cultural and other biases of scientific medicine, understanding how and in whose interest the system works, and assessing the natural role in which the patient is cast, are all basic elements of empowerment. To these, women have added several woman-centred, community-defined initiatives in health care practice. Such initiatives include, first of all, self-examination – an excellent tool in disease prevention and a technique for rediscovering and reappropriating one's body. Secondly, group learning adds a unique dimension of solidarity to health care education. Self-help groups provide mutual support to every member of the group. As well, self-help initiatives add an essentially political dimension to the actions undertaken. Women's self-help groups threaten the traditional medical system since they question both the sacred status of experts and the authoritarianism of health professionals of all kinds. Instead, the egalitarian relationships of self-help groups favour a greater sense of self, more autonomy, and better self-expression of laywomen whose knowledge is rooted in their life experience. Although these initiatives are enjoyed by a minority, government bureaucracies are trying to absorb them into their ways of doing things, their rules of the game, and thus may kill what was once so special about them. While this may be the price of success, it must be opposed. This, of course, is almost impossible to do without adequate financial resources!

Two other approaches empower women in health matters: women's health clinics and the various methods of feminist counselling and therapy. (The latter concept is much better expressed by the terms "feminist intervention," a neutral expression which does not suggest any special disciplinary definition or pathology.) These approaches, however, involve recourse to health professionals – usually women themselves. Although I have not seen any statistics on the question, it seems to me that the great majority of women I know are now choosing a female physician or specialist. A smaller number of women are also choosing to deal with health care through community clinics, and whenever possible, a women's health centre. (Most unfortunately, a stigma of poverty still attaches to such clinics.) In situations such as these, women feel more at ease; they trust these providers more. Nurse practitioners, even given the small number currently practicing in Canada, usually play a vital role in these settings. Feminist approaches and practices have also been developed for mental health care, for the victims of violence or sexual abuse, and for other social services.

A note in passing: none of these initiatives has a chance to succeed and expand until the fee schedule of our provincial health plans, which now only pays for physicians' services is revised and altered to accommodate other health practitioners. This alteration is, of course, made possible by the Canada Health Act (1984). At the same time, the concept of a fee for each medical procedure could also be reviewed to see if there might not be a better, more efficient means of ensuring well-being.

Earlier I mentioned female physicians, nurses, counsellors, therapists, social workers, and psychologists. While I believe that it is essential to focus on women as users of the health-care system, and as health providers *par excellence*, I also believe that we should be working with female health professionals who are already in the health care system. At a time when faculties of medicine are graduating classes in which more than half the students are women and when 80 per cent of the graduates of schools of pharmacy are women, one wonders how this feminization of the profession will affect the practice of health care. Will more female physicians change medicine? Nobody really knows yet. One thing, however, is certain: women will probably benefit from the united efforts of feminists and female health professionals. This challenge is with us now.

The second wave of feminism – our wave – is now nearly twenty years old. This is a very short time in terms of social change, and, particularly in Canada, many positive changes have taken place. Many of the barriers against women have been broken down and many opportunities have opened up. In the minds of many sincere citizens the motto now seems to be "the sky is the limit." Those of us who teach know that young girls and women refuse to discuss feminist issues since they believe that feminism is *passé* and that there are no problems anymore. But the truth is that our heightened expectations of women, by themselves and by others, has *added* to the so-called traditional roles and responsiblilities. Yes, some new sharing of housework is taking place among a number of young couples. For many families and for many women, however, this dream is still an illusion. The private sphere has remained private and so have the issues associated with it.

Until this situation changes, the health of women will suffer. The double roles and double workloads that our society now expects from women exhaust them. They are pulled in opposite directions by the excessive and conflicting demands of family and profession. Women are now not only in paid employment but also in training, in business and politics. Yet domestic tasks, physical or emotional, still fall to women as a matter of course. Women remain the ones with the ultimate responsibility for infants, children, and adolescents. They are now more and more the ones faced with the care of the old – the 75-, 80-, 85-year-old parent, mother-in-law, aunt, or cousin. By an incredible social lie, women and mothers are made to believe that it all comes down to a matter of good organization. If *she* is well organized, *she* can cope. Others did it before her. I denounce that mystification as the most serious threat to women's health and well-being. Women's health must be protected not only by the demedicalization of life and the empowerment of women but also by the entry of the private sphere into the political agenda.

NOTES

1 Originally presented as "Notes for an Opening Address" at the Eleventh Annual Conference of the Canadian Research Institute for the Advancement of Women.

2 Hon. Monique Bégin was Minister of National Health and Welfare from September 1977 to June 1979 and from March 1980 to September 1984.
3 This forum, held 29–31 Oct. 1987 and entitled "Maternity in the Laboratory," produced bilingual conference proceedings available under the title *Sortir la maternité du laboratoire*, Québec: Gouvernement du Québec/ Conseil du Statut de la femme, 1988.

REFERENCES

· Berliner, Howard S. 1984. "Scientific Medicine Since Flexner." In J. Warren Salmon, ed., *Alternative Medicines: Popular and Policy Perspectives*. New York: Tavistock.

Boston Women's Health Book Collective 1984. *Our Bodies, Ourselves*. New York: Simon and Schuster.

Essai sur la santé des femme 1981. Quebec City: Gouvernement du Québec, Conseil du statut de la femme.

Illich, Ivan 1976. *Medical Nemesis: The Expropriation of Health*. New York: Pantheon.

Ontario. Task Force on Implementation of Midwifery in Ontario 1987. *Report of the Task Force on Implementation of Midwivery in Ontario*. [Toronto]: Task Force on Implementation of Midwifery in Ontario.

ANDREA LEBOWITZ

Illness as Metaphor in the Nineteenth-Century Novel

Andrea Lebowitz explores the ways in which the authors of three nineteenth-century novels (*Persuasion* by Jane Austen, *Wuthering Heights* by Emily Brontë, and *Jane Eyre* by Charlotte Brontë) use health and illness to figure the condition of women in a patriarchal culture and manipulate these states to resist and condemn a society which infects its female members. Through illness, *Persuasion* represents the powerlessness of women legally and economically and cautions against the acceptance of male definitions; *Wuthering Heights* displays the ways in which a powerful heroine uses her health to resist confinement; and *Jane Eyre* demonstrates how "redundant" females are made sick and how acquiescence to society's definitions brings death.

La maladie comme métaphore dans les romans au dix-neuvième siècle

Andrea Lebowitz examine les manières dont trois romans du dix-neuvième siècle (*Persuasion* de Jane Austen, *Wuthering Heights* d'Emily Brontë et *Jane Eyre* de Charlotte Brontë) utilisent la santé et la maladie pour dépeindre la condition des femmes dans une culture patriarcale, et se servent de ces états comme moyen de résistance ou de condamnation d'une société qui attaque ses membres du sexe féminin. À l'aide de la maladie, *Persuasion* démontre l'absence de pouvoir juridique et économique des femmes, et met en garde contre l'acceptation des définitions masculines; *Wuthering Heights* montre de quelle façon une héroïne se sert de sa santé pour résister à l'enfermement; *Jane Eyre* démontre que l'inutilité sociale peut conduire à la maladie et que l'acceptation des définitions établies par la société peut mener à la mort.

On first looking into cultural representations of health and illness, we observe a constellation of attitudes: states of health are assigned moral value, patients are judged for and by their illness, and, finally, disease is used to define character. Sickness can also act as a source of desire, particularly when a frail, weak woman suffers from a "decorous" disease like consumption with its unnatural heightening of the bloom of youthful complexion. While sickness may make a woman more desirable, it can simultaneously define her as inferior, hence reducing the object of desire to manageable proportions. Conversely, health can be objectionable, especially when displayed by a lower-class woman or a woman who refuses to "do her duty" (English and Ehrenreich 1973).

In her essay *Illness as Metaphor*, Susan Sontag attempts to strip illness of these "lurid metaphors," but she achieves her end by surveying the range of, often contradictory, figurative meanings applied to physical and mental illness. Beginning with the equation between the illness and the character of the patient, Sontag identifies two hypotheses which expand the meaning of sickness. Social deviation is figured as illness, and conversely, illness reveals social disruption or malfunction. Secondly, all illness turns into a psychological manifestation in which the patient is responsible because she or he desires or deserves sickness. Ultimately the victim is blamed for being ill, and often the victim pays with a deserved death.

Although our cultural artefacts are littered with the dead bodies of powerful heroines who inspire a necrophiliac desire in their lovers and writers, I intend to look at the ways in which actual bodily illnesses are manipulated to reveal not only the heroine's state of physical health but also her moral and spiritual well-being, for, although feminist literary critics have paid close attention to the metaphoric meanings of mental disorders, somewhat less attention has been paid to bodily illness. Yet it too can serve writers as a code for representing states of being. In addition, we will see that, when women writers manipulate states of physical health, they may do so to warn or to challenge as well as to define. Unlike their brother writers, women use illness to reveal the nature *of an individual character* rather than the whole sex. In addition, women writers use sickness not to blame the patient but to condemn the society which infects the female characters. Unfettered by such a subtle vision of reality, male writers can write off half the species with a stroke of the pen or a stroke.

The three novels (*Persuasion* by Jane Austen, *Wuthering Heights* by Emily Brontë, and *Jane Eyre* by Charlotte Brontë) present an interesting range of ways in which illness can be manipulated to express differing aspects of the nature and condition of women. Through illness and accident, Austen defines the powerlessness of women legally and economically, cautions against the acceptance of male definitions of being, and signals the heroine's acquisition of power through her return to youthful health and vigour. While employing several of these strategies, Emily Brontë also displays the ways in which a powerful heroine uses her own health to resist confinement. Charlotte Brontë demonstrates how "redundant" females are literally made sick and also suggests that acquiescence to society's definitions returns a woman to a total state of nature, which is also a total silence and lack of control of culture.

Let us begin, then, with Jane Austen's last novel, *Persuasion*, which was published posthumously in 1818. Despite this date, the work appears to mirror the earlier Augustan sensibility, which recommended reason and balance in morals as well as manners. But all is not what it seems, for the supposed consensus is fractured and the social and moral worlds are in a kind of quiet chaos. In her article, Mary Poovey (1983) suggests that the heroine, Anne Elliot, is in fact the only moral person at the start of the novel. Rather than giving her power, her superiority of insight and education leaves Anne isolated and alienated from her surroundings, over which she has no control. Her situation is exacerbated by two further causes of confinement: her father, Sir Walter Elliot, a vain and self-important baronet, has gone so far into debt that the family is forced to decamp from the ancestral home, which now must be let to strangers in order to pay the bills. Further, Anne is trapped by her advanced age of twenty-eight. Her youth, health, and bloom gone,[1] she has little hope of escape through marriage or any other means. Eight years earlier, she had been persuaded to end her engagement to a young naval officer, Frederick Wentworth, because neither his position nor his parentage was thought suitable for the middle daughter of a minor aristocrat. In short, defined and confined by patriarchy, Anne no longer has value as a commodity on the marriage market and hence is a useless encumbrance to her irresponsbile father. Anne's condition is figured and reflected in, and contrasted to, that of other female characters, particularly Louisa Musgrove, the new young love interest of Frederick, and Mrs. Smith, a poor, paralyzed widow who has neither money nor friends although she was once a gentleman's daughter.[2]

At first glance Louisa appears to be the antithesis of Anne because the younger woman is healthy, vigorous, and apparently determined and decisive. But Louisa's true character and situation are exposed when she meets with an accident of her own making. As Louisa and her companions walk about Lyme, she insists on being "jumped down" from the upper Cobb to the lower walkway. Although Wentworth fears that she might harm herself, he agrees to catch her and does so on the first jump. But Louisa rushes back up and again launches herself into space, this time before Wentworth can persuade her to stop or prepare to break her fall. Instead she crashes to the pavement and is taken up with no outward injury but unconscious from the blow to her head. Clearly the injury which leaves no mark but renders her speechless, senseless, and unconscious suggests that she is not a free personality but a captive trying to "win" a man by aping his behaviour. Conversely, Anne acts decisively and with authority. She alone keeps her wits during the accident and directs the operations to get Louisa medical help. Frederick, incapacitated by his sense of guilt, recognizes that he remains unchanged in his love for Anne and that his courting of Louisa has been a cruel charade. Despite his realization, Frederick is tied and confined, since everyone assumes that he is engaged to Louisa, although this has never taken place. In other words, his unthinking behaviour has not only allowed harm to befall Louisa but tied him to her, since he cannot now abandon her and hope to win Anne.[3] The plot is apparently at an impasse. Only a redirection of Louisa's affections can release Wentworth.

While there is a suitor in the wings, his attraction to Louisa is as remarkable to the characters in the novel as it is to the reader. Captain Benwick, another naval man, has recently lost his fiancée, Fanny Harville. A rather melancholy man, Benwick has brought his grief to the Harville family, and they comfort and support him in their mutual loss. It is thus with shock and amazement that the Harvilles watch Benwick court and propose to the semi-invalid Louisa. His inconstancy to Fanny and the ease with which he turns his love to Louisa appall them. But what of this love? It seems that here we have a rather classic example of desire inspired by the frail, sickly woman. Benwick turns from his dead love to one recently near to death, and most interestingly he woos her and recreates her through literature. Previous to her accident, Louisa had no time for books. Benwick could discuss his passion for the works of Byron and Sir Walter Scott only with Anne.[4] But in the passivity consequent to her accident, Louisa not only reads these texts but becomes Benwick's text. In short, he recreates her in his own image and writes her into his script of the melancholic literary lover. We can now see in hindsight that the previous Louisa had been another literary production, an image created to mirror her conception of the hearty, vigorous Wentworth. True determination and clarity have been Anne's, not Louisa's.

While Wentworth is being unshackled from his unwanted attachment to Louisa, Anne has moved on to visit the new establishment

of her father and sister in the city of Bath. It is here that she comes
into contact wth Mrs. Smith, a rediscovered old school friend, who,
with her anonymous name, is not only a double to Anne but also
the cautionary image at the heart of the novel. Mrs. Smith's physical
condition of paralysis obviously represents her condition as a redundant, unwanted, powerless woman. Her situation is worsened
by the fact that there is a possibility of realizing some money from
an investment her husband had, but the executor, a Mr. Elliot, who
is none other than the nearest male kin to Sir Walter Elliot, will do
nothing to help her to pursue this claim. Without health or funds,
she cannot act for herself. Silenced and immobilized, Mrs. Smith
clings with determination to her mental health. While some readers
might find this display of fortitude implausible, it seems important
for it clearly indicates that the cause of her situation rests not in her
nature but her situation. While Anne cannot offer Mrs. Smith mon-
etary or legal assistance, she does offer loyalty and support and
persists in visiting the sick woman, despite Sir Walter Elliot's con-
demnation and scorn that his daughter is wasting her time on a mere
nobody rather than pursuing important and fashionable people.
However, such female loyalty is rewarded.

Mr. Elliot, who rejected his family in his youth, has returned to
court them. Now a rich widower, he seeks status to burnish his riches.
He is apparently reformed, for he recognizes the superiority of
Anne. While she can find nothing in his manner to condemn him,
Anne experiences dis-ease about him and his obvious intentions to
propose to her. Confirmation of the correctness of her feelings comes
from Mrs. Smith, who has documentary proof that Mr. Elliot is not
what he seems. His refusal to assist her demonstrates that he possesses neither loyalty nor compassion.

The stage is now set for the reunion of Anne and Wentworth.
Anne precipitates the situation by allowing her conversation to be
overheard by Frederick. Engaged with Captain Harville in a discussion of Benwick's inconstancy to Fanny and the more general
topic of who are more faithful, men or women, Anne asserts her
loyalty by arguing that the condition of women makes them more
constant and that the fickleness of women is a male myth perpetuated
by the control men have of literary texts. By this act of seizing language from male control, Anne restores herself and Frederick to
health and happiness.

While Anne's restoration to health of mind and body is gradual,
Catherine's decline in *Wuthering Heights* is sharp, swift, and ultimately
brought on by her own hand. In turning to Emily Brontë's novel we
have moved forward to the year 1847 and a very different world.

Surrounded as she and her family were by the patriarchal presence of their father Patrick, the wild beauty and cruelty of the landscape of the moors, and the social revolt of groups like the Luddites, Emily was early acquainted with rebellion and discontent as well as the imaginative escape offered by literary creation.

Catherine's first words come to us through a makeshift diary, written in the blank margins of a Bible. These words are "'An awful Sunday! ... I wish my father were back again. Hindley is a detestable substitute — his conduct to Heathcliff is atrocious — H. and I are going to rebel — we took our initiatory step this evening'" (Brontë 1965, 62). This attempt at rebellion continues throughout, and when Catherine can no longer rebel in life, she rebels through death.

One notable way in which this novel differs from *Persuasion* is in its emphasis on childhood, which (like her brother Romantics) Emily sees as a time of freedom. Isolated from the demands of society in the aerie of the Heights, young Catherine finds her heaven on the rock of the moors and in the flint of her other half, the foundling Heathcliff. That they are male and female who together form a unity beyond gender confinement or class restriction seems obvious. But they are also girl and boy, and although in youth they are "half savage and hardy and free" (Catherine's words as she is dying and wishing again to be her younger self), biology as scripted by the conventions of nineteenth century patriarchy overwhelms them.

The edenic world of childhood, so important to the lives of the characters, shatters with the death of the father and his replacement by Catherine's older brother Hindley. Returning with a frail, ladylike wife, who has tuberculosis but is seen to be the epitome of womanly beauty, he alters the children's world. Class and gender are imposed. Heathcliff is banished to the stables, deprived of education, and separated for the first time from Catherine. She is coerced by flattery and attention and the accoutrements of a lady. Although quite clearly Hindley's wife suffers from the confinement of decorous ladyhood, she attempts to infect Catherine with the same social malady. The children scorn both force and flattery and seek to remain together. Banished from the fire with its connotations of civilization, the children plan their revolt. On the fateful night recorded in her diary, Catherine and Heathcliff sneak from the house and run down to the Grange. This is the home of the local magistrate and chief family of the district. Looking through a window, the youngsters are beguiled by the ornamentation and splendour of the interior. They laugh at the petted Linton brother and sister who are fighting over a small lapdog. But not all the dogs at the Grange are harmless bits of fluff. Alarmed by the noise, the servants release a powerful bulldog named Skulker, who seizes and wounds Catherine. When he is finally dragged off, the dog's "huge, purple tongue [is] hanging half a foot out of his mouth, and his pendant lips [are] streaming with bloody slaver" (Brontë 1965, 90). That this figures a sexual seizure and assault hardly needs comment. When the Lintons recognize Catherine, they take her into the deceiving interior of their home and drive off Heathcliff. Although the Lintons give Catherine medical attention, they also completely immobilize her in a large invalid chair. Her initiation into the world of class and gender has been achieved in a maiming ritual.

Power is now on the side of society. Hindley further abuses Heathcliff and turns him more and more into a beast of burden. The Linton boy, Edgar, inspired and infatuated by Catherine's vitality, pursues her despite his obvious alarm at her temper, which occasionally escapes her control. Caught in between, Catherine "adopt[s] a double character without exactly intending to deceive any one" (Brontë 1965, 107). Refusing to abandon Heathcliff, yet recognizing that escape from Hindley may only be possible through Edgar, she tries to straddle two worlds, for she is now and always a non-negotiating heroine.

With Edgar's proposal, a choice seems forced. Catherine tries to discuss her dilemma with Nelly, the housekeeper, who, although unsympathetic, is the only confidant available. On the one hand, Catherine wishes to become Mrs. Linton, for she will be the first lady in the neighbourhood, and even more importantly, she will escape the madhouse the Heights has become since the death of Hindley's wife after the birth of their first child. Yet Catherine also feels that although she should not abandon Heathcliff, marriage with him is impossible and would "degrade" her, since he has been brought so low by Hindley. Nelly has become aware of Heathcliff's presence in the room but does not tell Catherine, and he rushes out before hearing the end of Catherine's words, which assert that she will use her future husband's money to rescue Heathcliff for she cannot possibly exist without him. While Nelly and many critics after her have dismissed Catherine's assertions, I take them quite seriously as an indication of Catherine's desire to transcend convention and to have both worlds. I do not see the statement as a rationalization, and if it reveals naïveté, it is born of Catherine's ignorance of the world, not of her bad faith. However, Heathcliff disappears, and Catherine spends the whole night in vigil. Drenched by rain, she is ill by morning and is overcome in both body and mind. Catherine, half savage and hardy and free, falls into illness when she is separated from herself, alienated from herself by the demands of class and gender.

Three years pass, during which Catherine and Edgar marry. Life at the Grange resembles the calm before the storm, which breaks out with the return of Heathcliff, who has somehow (and it is never explained, except perhaps by the very fact that he has grown to manhood) gained both education and money. Initially Catherine cajoles her husband into allowing Heathcliff to visit. This temporary truce is broken by Edgar's jealousy and his fear that Heathcliff will attempt to revenge himself by seducing Edgar's sister Isabella. When Edgar demands that Catherine choose between him and Heathcliff, she locks herself in her room and refuses food. Scorning Edgar, who seeks solace in the library, patriarchy's stronghold, Catherine seeks to escape from her own body, which she calls a "shattered prison." Realizing that there is no way to resist her marriage and the forthcoming birth of a child, or to put it conversely, there is no way to keep Heathcliff, her healthy, vigorous half or other self, she chooses death rather than capitulation. Her self-starvation, fever, and death present different meanings to readers. Some see it as childish petulance, others as anorexia nervosa, still others as a hunger strike. There is much in a name, for each term suggests a very different interpretative meaning. Is she a child unwilling to face adult responsibility, a neurotic adolescent, or a political prisoner using the only means of resistance – her own body? To opt for a reading which sees her as a child demanding everything dismisses the whole symbolic importance of health in the novel. Whenever the characters are free of restrictions, they are vigorous and healthy. Once ensnared, they sicken mentally and physically. Thus, when Catherine recognizes that she can no longer get back to that state of freedom – that is, when she recognizes that marriage and maternity have claimed her body, she escapes by her own hand rather than capitulate to a state of complete imprisonment and illness.

Emily's sister Charlotte in her novel *Jane Eyre* (1847) creates another rebellious heroine, but Charlotte also attempts to create a plot that will accommodate rebellion in life. Beginning as a poor, plain orphan, Jane is completely marginalized and seems to have received three deadly strikes. Yet she survives to achieve fortune, acknowledgement of her mental and moral superiority, and family. In doing so, she has to resist many things, including ill health. Unlike Catherine, Jane is not forced to employ the ultimate resistance of death; indeed, to accept death is to capitulate, as does her childhood friend Helen Burns, another cautionary double.

As an unwanted foundling in her aunt's home, Jane's first act of rebellion is rewarded by imprisonment in the famous red room. No longer willing to accommodate the irksome foster child, Jane's aunt sends her off to a charity school that specializes in educating poor

girls to their proper place. Lowood School enforces strict codes of
dress and behaviour and allows the girls no ornament of personal
adornment and very little physical or intellectual pleasure. Run by
a sadistic minister, the Reverend Mr. Brocklehurst, the school keeps
the girls in a physical state of near starvation, worsened by insufficient heating and inadequate clothing. That the students fall prey
to an epidemic of typhus is certainly understandable, but it also
suggests that these poor girls are redundant and unwanted. At best
they will be serviceable, but society would do better yet to simply
dispose of them without added expense. Although Jane is not infected by the disease, she is tempted by the self-immolation of her
little friend, Helen Burns. This child, although intellectually gifted
and morally acute, accepts the school's vision of her as an unrepen-
tant, undisciplined sinner. When overcome by sickness, Helen wel-
comes death as an escape from her own infected nature. Jane is torn
between her love for Helen and her resistance against Helen's acquiescence to society's definitions.

Although Brocklehurst is removed and conditions improve,
Lowood can offer only temporary shelter and happiness. At eighteen, Jane moves on to become the governess of Mr. Rochester's ward,
Adele. With this job, Jane seems to have achieved more than any
poor single woman could hope for: a well-paying position in an
establishment where she is neither overworked nor demeaned. Yet
she remains unsatisfied and longs for a fuller, freer life. One avenue
to this life seems to be offered by Mr. Rochester. After her impas-
sioned assertion that she is his equal, he offers marriage. Yet this is
not to be, for not only does he have a wife but he also seeks to
ensnare Jane, to keep her like a resident of a seraglio and adorn her
with the foreign trappings of a lady. As in her relationship to Helen,
Jane is torn between resistance and capitulation to Rochester's need
and desire. After a night filled with dreams of maternal figures
urging her to flee, Jane leaves Thornfield.

Perhaps the most problematic section of the novel follows. Once
more on the road, Jane "inadvertently" leaves her money and pos-
sessions behind in the coach, and is cast homeless and without resources or friends in a foreign landscape. Her self-punishment seems
to be the reaction to her self-determination, a self-imposed suffering
for having refused to accept male desire. In her wanderings, she
reacts to nature as to a welcoming mother and asserts that nature
at least will give her repose. But nature is no answer and offers
neither comfort nor safety.

As Margaret Homans (1983) has suggested, acquiescence to nature
will be the final triumph of culture over Jane, who will be completely

separated from her quest to conquer culture's restrictions. Again Jane resists and forces herself back into society. Having discovered her unknown family, the Rivers, she at last finds home and soon receives fortune, yet one temptation to accept society's definition of women remains (Rich 1979). Inspired by St. John Rivers's religious passion, Jane comes close to accepting his offer that she join him as a missionary to India. Only one condition deters her, for he insists that they venture forth as husband and wife, despite his obvious passionate love for another woman whom he feels to be unworthy of his mission. Jane refuses complete capitulation and pictures this proposed marriage as a physical as well as a mental death.

Her resistance to St. John is solidified when she hears Rochester's call and returns to him. Now a widower and maimed in his attempt to save Bertha, his insane wife who finally escaped to destroy herself and Rochester's house, Thornfield, Rochester acknowledges his pride and former desire to entrap Jane. And so reader, she married him, and therein hangs a debate. Does Jane finally give up her quest and accept the closure of marriage, or does Brontë try to envision an ending which goes beyond the conventional ending, which allows the rebellious quest to continue? While this debate cannot be resolved in a sentence and will probably never be resolved except in each reader's mind, it does seem important to note that the pattern of sickness and health which has informed the conflict between acquiescence and resistance is brought into the coda of the book. Not only does Jane exert her own power and health but she is also able to restore some of Rochester's lost health. Conversely, St. John Rivers quickly dies in his Indian mission.

While all of these characters (and their authors) are by no means free of the infection of patriarchal definitions, they do resist and rebel and attempt to subvert the dominant ideology, often through a manipulation of states of physical health and sickness. In conclusion, it seems that there is ample evidence to support the suggestion that states of physical health can be used to represent the condition of women, to warn against that condition, or to expose the very nature of gender definitions.

NOTES

1 The female condition is often represented by horticultural images, which are another way of indicating an alignment between women and nature.
2 Anne's younger married sister Mary is a type of woman found in several Austen novels. Without sense or control, she constantly harps on the state

of her nerves and the condition of her health. This hypochondria clearly represents her mental and moral condition.

3 This situation of two women who present real and imaginary love to the hero is a way of demonstrating his growth toward maturity and sensibility, signalled by his recognition of the superior woman. This movement can be compared to the heroine's reaction to two suitors, discussed by Kennerd (1978).

4 Several key passages in the book occur as literary discussions. It would seem after all that literary criticism can affect the world.

REFERENCES

Austen, Jane 1818/1965. *Persuasion*, ed. D.W. Harding. Harmondsworth: Penguin.

Brontë, Charlotte 1847/1953. *Jane Eyre*. Harmondsworth: Penguin.

Brontë, Emily 1847/1965. *Wuthering Heights*, ed. David Daiches. Harmondsworth: Penguin.

English, Deirdre and Barbara Ehrenreich 1973. *Complaints and Disorders: The Sexual Politics of Sickness*. Old Westbury: Feminist Press.

Kennard, Jean 1978. *Victims of Convention*. Hamden, Conn.: Archon Books.

Homans, Margaret 1983. "Dreaming of Children: Literalization in *Jane Eyre* and *Wuthering Heights*." In Juliann E. Fleenor, ed., *The Female Gothic*. Montreal/London: Eden Press.

Poovey, Mary 1983. "*Persuasion* and the Promises of Love." In Caroline G. Heilbrun and Margaret R. Higonnet, eds., *The Representation of Women*. Baltimore: Johns Hopkins University Press.

Rich, Adrienne 1979. "Jane Eyre: Temptations of a Motherless Woman." In A. Rich, *On Lies, Secrets and Silence*. New York: Norton.

DAWN CURRIE

Women's Liberation and Women's Mental Health: Towards a Political Economy of Eating Disorders

Current increases in anorexia are a telling indictment of the lack of well-being of women in affluent industrialized nations. The prevalence of the psychoanalytic notion that anorexics are rejecting femininity through deliberately arrested physical development is particularly discouraging in that it encourages intervention at the individual level. In this regard, feminist approaches represent an advance since they emphasize cultural prescriptions for thinness, shifting intervention from the individual to the social realm. At the same time, however, Currie (1988) maintains that cultural approaches are inadequate,because they do not differentiate between the reproduction of culture and the conditions and relations of its production. For this reason, cultural approaches are not able to explain class patterns of anorexia: while all women are exposed to the sociocultural pressures towards thinness, those from middle-class professional families are selectively at risk. This article explores the development of a materialist approach that better fits the empirical description and that links the struggle for womem's mental health to that for a transformation of the material – rather than strictly cultural – conditions of existence.

La libération des femmes et la santé mentale des femmes: vers une approche politique et économique des désordres nutritionnels

L'actuelle recrudescence de l'anorexie est un phénomène qui remet en question le mieux-être des femmes dans les sociétés industrielles dites "d'abondance". La prédominance de l'analyse psychanalytique selon laquelle les anorexiques rejettent leur féminité en arrêtant délibérement leur développement physique, est particulièrement inquiétante en ce sens que cette vision encourage l'intervention uniquement au niveau individuel. À cet égard, la perspective féministe représente un pas en avant en attirant plutôt l'attention sur les pressions culturelles prescrivant la min-

ceur comme taille idéale. À ce sujet, Currie soutient toutefois que les
approches basées exclusivement sur le rôle joué par la culture sont inadé-
quates, car elles n'établissent pas la différence entre la reproduction de la
culture d'une part et les conditions et les relations impliquées dans sa
production d'autre part. C'est pour cette raison que les approches culturelles ne peuvent expliquer le rôle de la classe sociale dans les modèles de
comportement: alors que toutes les femmes sont exposées aux pressions
socio-culturelles prescrivant la minceur, les femmes provenant de familles
professionnelles de classe moyenne sont plus sujettes que les autres à
l'anorexie. Dans cet article, Currie tente de développer une approche ma-
térialiste qui reflète davantage la description empirique et qui suggère
que la lutte des femmes pour contrôler leur santé mentale doit d'abord
passer par la transformation matérielle – et non pas seulement culturelle
– des conditions de leur existence.

Part of the current trend of being fashionably thin, anorexia refers
to the practice of dieting to the point of self-starvation. In Canada,
this disorder afflicts primarily young women, particularly those from
professional families.[1] In 1986, researchers reported that the twin
eating disorders of anorexia nervosa and bulimia have increased in
frequency sixfold or more since 1983 (Toronto *Globe and Mail*,
26 October 1986).[2] At the same time, little progress has been made
in the treatment of this disease. Therapists report that, overall, less
than half (40 per cent) of anorexics are cured in a global sense, while
approximately 30 per cent are significantly improved but continue
to lead symptomatic or impaired lives. Of the 9 per cent of diagnosed
anorexics who die from causes related to their condition, suicide is
the leading cause of death (Thompson and Gans 1985, 292–3). Given
this dismal record, the individualistic orientation underlying traditional approaches is being challenged by models which include social
causes of anorexia.

Feminist writings in particular explore the importance of cultural
factors, emphasizing the media stereotyping of women. They point
out that, since the 1960s, portrayals of the ideal body weight for
women emphasize thinness, and the idealized woman is the long-
legged pre-adolescent (Schwartz *et al.* 1985). A number of studies
have documented this preference for greater thinness through evaluations of *Playboy* centrefolds, assessments of contestants and win-
ners of Miss America Pageants, and public opinion surveys about
"the most beautiful women of the world." Since 1970, Elizabeth Tay-
lor has fallen in the polls as the ideal woman, replaced by Twiggy,
who ranked number one in 1976 (Schwartz *et al.* 1985, 97). Within

the feminist literature, therefore, the notion prevalent in traditional theories that anorectics are rejecting femininity through deliberately arrested physical development has been replaced by an emphasis on their overconformity. Writers point out that dieting is a widespread practice among healthy North American women, carried out for cosmetic rather than health reasons.[3] After polling subscribers in 1984, *Glamour* reported that the majority of respondents were either dissatisfied with or ashamed of their stomach, hips, or thighs (Boskind-White 1985, 114). From this perspective, anorexics are portrayed as being obsessed with cultural prescriptions for thinness which include harsh judgements of fat women.

INTERVENTION AS CULTURAL REVOLUTION: THE PROBLEM OF IDEALISM

By drawing attention to the devalued position of women in our society as a causal factor in anorexia, feminist perspectives link anorexia specifically, and women's mental health generally, to issues of power. But although recent writings highlight eating disorders as gender linked, the insights provided have not been adequately explored. I believe that this failure is rooted in the idealism of current feminist approaches. By idealism I mean that they portray consciousness as a mere reflection of prevalent cultural stereotypes and values. As a consequence, change is advocated at the symbolic level of cultural representation, or as cultural revolution. The problem is that this perspective fails to differentiate between the reproduction of culture and the conditions and relations of its production. Focusing narrowly on the ways in which women internalize cultural images and values, material differences between women have not been addressed. Class differences in the frequency of anorexia have not been explained. While all women are exposed to the sociocultural pressures towards thinness, those from middle-class professional families are at the greatest risk of developing eating disorders. To date, these class differences have not been explained, unless it can be argued that socialization practices vary according to social class.

A second problem of idealism concerns the identification of new cultural stereotypes of women as the root of the problem. Bennett and Gurin (1982, 171), for example, argue that the new media image of women is symbolic of Women's Liberation: against traditional images of women as either sexual or maternal objects, the liberated woman is portrayed as athletic rather than physically passive, androgynously independent, and characterized by a nonreproductive sexuality. Feminists struggling against old cultural portrayals of women therefore are faced with the issue of whether images with these more positive connotations are simply resulting in a new disease for women. Analysis again shifts away from the structures of patriarchy and class, this time towards the Women's Liberation Movement, so that researchers like Johnson (1986) claim that the feminist movement is causally linked to the current epidemic of eating disorders.[4]

Given these problems this paper will sketch out a dialectical framework which includes the production of cultural meanings – the externalization of societal values – as well as internalization of these meanings. Not only will we be able to develop a theoretical approach which better fits the empirical description, but this approach will also direct us to interventions at the material, rather than strictly cultural, level of the struggle for women's emancipation.

WOMEN AS OTHER: THE LEGACY OF SIMONE DE BEAUVOIR

As a critique of the Aristotlean tradition and from an existentialist perspective outlined by Sartre, de Beauvoir argues that consciousness itself has no content; consciousness can only be consciousness of something. This something is discovered through an active relation to the material world. For this reason, Sartre distinguishes between a thing as existing in-itself and consciousness as existing for-itself. The being of a thing is simply "what it is." Being in the nonconscious world represents a "fullness such that each thing is absolutely identical with itself, and no more total plenitude can be imagined" (Sartre 1969, 74). The being in-itself requires nothing beyond itself. On the other hand, the being for-itself lacks the fullness of being that things have, so that it strives for the completeness of the thing in-itself. That is to say, the for-itself desires to give itself being, to justify its own existence. However, consciousness does not strive to be a thing. Rather, it desires the impossible union of the for-itself and in-itself: to exist as God. Because the for-itself can never reach this state of union with being in-itself, consciousness lies in its relational character to objects of consciousness without being identical to them. In short, consciousness can never take on an identity or essence in the manner that things have identities or essences. Consciousness is free to be anything, while at the same time, it is nothing except this freedom. Whatever meaning human consciousness acquires, it does so through action or labour. For both Sartre and de Beauvoir, one is simply what one does. Actions or labour are externalization of what one is. Hence if, as de Beauvoir herself later says, a woman does little, then she is little. To be therefore requires self-affirming activity.

Although consciousness realizes itself through action as giving meaning to its existence, the range of possible actions is not infinite. Sartre claims that in an attempt to approximate union between for-itself and in-itself, consciousness has a tendency to see itself as identical with the actions or roles it chooses. Through identification, one no longer has to continually give meaning to one's life; the role which one chooses is believed to be sufficient to justify one's existence. Because this is an explicit denial of one's freedom and the responsibility which accompanies this freedom, Sartre calls this "bad faith." Once one adopts a role in bad faith, it is not necessary for consciousness to make the kind of continued decisions that "authentic" humans make because the role itself determines what is possible and what is not. The role or activity gives the person a sense of being something concrete. Furthermore, society reinforces this type of identification so that both men and women can lead an unauthentic existence. However, as de Beauvoir goes on to explore, the consciousness of men and women is differentially developed.

While consciousness defines itself in relation to objects of consciousness, the social world is constituted by more than mere objects: in the social world, objects of consciousness include other human beings. Because consciousness is nothing apart from its object, it becomes human only when the object of consciousness is another human being. In short, consciousness *is*, only in so far as it has an object and is human, only in so far as the object is human. This is what Sartre calls being for-others: existence as Object in the consciousness of another Subject. De Beauvoir argues that being for-others epitomizes women's status as the "second sex." In a patriarchal society, man defines himself as different from and against woman as "other," an object in his world. However, to seek recognition as a human being is a desire to be recognized as a conscious and creative being and not as a mere object in the world. As long as women are given recognition as a mere body or thing, they are not recognized as self-conscious human beings. Recognized merely as sex objects, their value is tied solely to the body and their worth is not truly human worth. Denied entry to the world in which consciousness is affirmed through socially valued labour, as primarily wives and mothers, women are affirmed by their relation to men – never *vice versa*. On the everyday level, men assume the role of Subject, women that of Object. As such, women's nature is not defined through self-affirming labour. Rather, at both the material level of activity and the cultural level of symbolic order, it is men who define women's potential, and they do so in a way which prevents women from becoming autonomous Subjects.

WOMEN AS OTHER: CONSTRUCTING SELF AS ANOREXIC

While there are a number of problems with an existentialist approach,[5] for our purposes *The Second Sex* is useful in that it locates the development of women's consciousness within the context of their material as well as cultural world. Specifically, women develop a sense of self through roles which relegate them to being for-others. However, de Beauvoir herself notes that existing as "other" – as Object rather than as Subject – is not an eternal and irrevocable condition, as implied by many writers (see for example Ortner 1972). Rather, the ways in which women are denied authenticity are a consequence of relations specific to a given class in a given society. From this perspective, processes specific to advanced capitalist societies can be identified as historical and material preconditions of the construction of the self as anorexic.

For de Beauvoir, it is through the roles of wife and mother that women perpetually exist primarily for-others. Focusing on marriage, she notes that while it is true that the two sexes are necessary to each other, this necessity has never brought a condition of reciprocity. While marriage may be seen as a burden and a benefit for men and women alike, for women marriage is the only means of acquiring identity, of being integrated into the community (de Beauvoir 1953, 402). In contrast, a man is socially an independent and complete individual; he is regarded first of all in terms of the work he does for the collective – in capitalist societies his employment. The rhetoric of Women's Liberation notwithstanding, opportunities for women outside marriage remain restricted, so that women's futures continue to be linked to men.

While it is true that women's rates of participation in the labour force have increased, the types of jobs held by women overall have not changed substantially. The majority of working women in Canada are found in service and clerical jobs, with professional careers largely restricted to the traditionally feminine ones in health care and teaching. Even within these professions women seldom hold the prestigious jobs. In 1984, only 8 per cent of employed women were in managerial or administrative positions (Advisory Council on the Status of Women). Canadian women remain concentrated in a female ghetto where chances for promotion are few and wages low.

In 1987, for every dollar a full-time male employee earned, a full-time female employee earned about 64 cents. In this way, marriage remains important to women's economic survival, while ideologies of romantic love and personal fulfillment obscure the nature of marriage as an economic institution (Leonard 1980). The few women who do not need marriage financially, therefore, are quite likely still to want to be married. For this reason, Baker (1985) reports that three quarters of Canadian adolescent girls dream of husbands in well-paid professions, suggesting that they see their future primarily as dependent on the better wages of men. Despite the so-called demise of marriage through increasing family breakdown, the reality is that most women continue to marry or remarry and have children, so that the current cultural emphasis upon singlehood reflects deferral and divorce rather than rejection of marriage and motherhood. In summary, women's future remains linked to men.

As objects of male conquest in both fantasy and reality, women have been and continue to be valued for physical beauty (Greer 1970; Cottin-Pogrebin 1983). This requires that, from adolescence onwards, women spend a lot of time (as well as money) learning and practicing how to be attractive; women literally work on their body image. At a time when both boys and girls become aware of their bodies, adolescence can introduce anxiety about appearance. For boys, body awareness is expressed as concern for physical strength and prowess – attributes which can be affirmed through activities such as sports – and popularity is associated with strength and athletic skills (Richmond-Abbott 1983). During the same period, girls focus upon physical beauty, which they believe to be crucial for popularity with boys. According to researchers, their perceptions are correct; physical attractiveness is rated much more highly as a desired characteristic of a date by boys than it is for girls (Wakil 1974; Center 1975; Cottin-Pogrebin 1983). When Bersheid and Walster (1974) presented males with photos of possible dates in which the physical attractiveness and probability of being accepted varied, subjects opted for the more attractive date regardless of the probability of acceptance. Furthermore, reported satisfaction with the date was a positive function of how attractive the date was. It is not surprising, therefore, that during adolescence women begin to report dissatisfaction with their bodies; as many as 60 per cent express a desire to change the way they look (Richmond-Abbott 1983, 160). At the same time, intellectual achievements are perceived as unfeminine,[6] so that this emerging body anxiety may become especially acute for academically successful girls. Despite current emphasis upon educational encouragement for women, girls who excel academically or harbour nontraditional aspirations receive "double messages," reflecting the reality that domestic roles and motherhood are still "on the agenda" (Sutherland 1978). Rather than providing women with avenues for self- fulfillment, therefore, academic success may increase girls' anxiety by undermining their acceptance by those who have been identified as necessary to their futures.

While it is true that both the media and the market now emphasize physical competence for both men and women, in the long run, popularized exercise programs such as Jane Fonda's Workout may simply exacerbate the "problem of the body."[7] Although the terms "health" and "self concept" have been associated with these types of workout programs, Szekely (1987b and c) argues that the programs define health as thinness. As a consequence, health has not only been associated with exercise but also with a plethora of consumer goods – "lean cuisine," "low-cal desserts," appetite curbs, exercise machinery – that may, in fact, have little to do with physical well-being (Szekely 1987b, 2). In this way, the current proliferation of fitness clubs, tanning clinics, weight-loss programs, home exercise kits, health foods, and the like does not suggest liberation from the tyranny of body imagery. On the contrary, the new image of women's bodies merely re-emphasizes the importance of physical rather than spiritual attributes. Furthermore, personal style is no longer limited to makeup, dress, and hairstyle. If the experts of the beauty and health industries are to be believed, body size and shape are now amenable to direct intervention.[8] For this reason, Szekely (1987b) argues that body shape is currently portrayed and experienced as a matter of personal choice. Normalcy, health, and beauty are the promised rewards of one's decision to exercise more and eat less. From personal interviews with women caught in the relentless pursuit of thinness, Szekely reports that women perceived difficulties or failure to achieve these goals as an individual failure of will. "Choice" and "self control" were two terms that these women used repeatedly to describe the meaning of being thin (Szekely 1987b, 8). The other side of the coin, of course, is the equation of body fat with personal inadequacy. Both women themselves and society generally equate being fat with the lack of self-discipline, slothfulness, and incompetency (Chernin 1982). In this way, a general body anxiety is transformed into feelings of guilt, reflected in the shame which many women report for having let themselves go. Due to this sense of personal responsibility, the body becomes an object of labour for many women. Given that few bodies can be willfully transformed into current cultural ideals, the relationship which many women feel towards their bodies is an antagonistic one, reflecting a conceptual separation between consciousness of self and body.

In summary, while the autonomy so recently ascribed to the new woman reflects actual changes in the material position of women, in reality rather than rhetoric, the opportunities now open to women remain the domain of the privileged few (Szekely 1987*b*). The glorified image of the new career woman is not a realistic aspiration for most Canadian women. For most, there are few real alternatives to traditional roles. However, for adolescent women from success-oriented families that can and do encourage their daughters academically, the double messages may render the transition from pre-pubescent emotional and economic dependency to the autonomy of adulthood problematic. For these women, the idealized image of the liberated career woman *is* accessible. Yet at the same time, its achievement is undermined by processes which continue to reproduce traditional role expectations for women. However, because the reproduction of social inequalities in capitalist society is submerged beneath the appearance of democratic opportunity, the nature of these contradictory messages will not be immediately apparent, so that ensuing conflict is directed inwards. Women individually cannot control the contradictory imagery constructed externally and symbolically. They can, however, struggle to control their personal body image. As Orbach (1986), Szekely (1987*a*), and others have documented through experiential approaches, the struggle of the anorexic is not simply to achieve thinness, but to achieve *control*. Thus the inward struggle of the anorexic can be reinterpreted as representing the internalization of conflict fostered by contradictions between the rhetoric and the reality of women's liberation in class society (Currie 1988).

RE-EXAMINING THE ROLE OF ADVERTISING

As a cultural phenomenon, the separation of self and body is rooted in material processes which create a disjunction between consciousness and the products of human labour that constitute material and cultural reality. Analyzing this disjunction as "commodity fetishism," Marx began with the production of commodities through alienated wage labour. Although commodities are produced by human labour, under capitalist production systems labour is not a self-affirming activity because it does not give expression to the authentic ideas, needs, and subjectivity of the labourer. Due to the separation of mental and manual work, labour is an activity which gives expression to the ideas of others. The continuity between subjectivity as conscious need and objects of labour as externalization of that need is severed. Commodities as objects of human labour are reunited with their makers through the mechanisms of the market, a process through which commodities stand above and against their makers. Rather than labourers determining the fate of the products of their labour, through their purchase commodities determine the quality of life of the workers: products of labour control their makers, rather than *vice versa*. The material world of commodities acquires a life of its own, but the social conditions and relations of production through which this inversion occurs is obscured and mystified. In the final analysis, social relations between humans appear as relations between things, while relations between commodities assume the character of social relations. As Goffman (1976) and others have argued, the purpose of advertising is to naturalize these relations, especially through the use of gender as a cultural theme.

In North American society, consumption is the activity whereby individuals partake in their social community. As we have seen, however, this community consists of relationships both between individuals and between individuals and the products of human labour. As the existential conditions of our existence, relations of consumption play a central role in the development of our conscious (as well as unconscious) being, particularly through the cultural sphere of advertising as a process whereby our desires, values, and sense of self are shaped. Advertising sets standards of femininity and instructs women as to the acquisition of this ideal through consumption. By investing products with the human quality of femininity, the message is that through the consumption of that product, the consumer becomes more feminine. However, advertising entails much more than the instruction of women: it is characterized by a more general objectification of women's bodies. The sexuality of women's bodies specifically is a central attribute given to commodities. This practice of associating women's bodies with inanimate objects is so widespread as almost not to require mention. The effect of such a practice is to transform women's bodies into symbols of consumption at both the ideological and real, practical level. The result of such advertising is that women live in a world where they confront their bodies as things outside themselves. The frequency of dieting, as well as observation at the everyday level, reveals the extent to which women feel uncomfortable in an authentic body, one which has not been transformed through depilation, deodorizing, reshaping, and so forth, for such a body is unfeminine. The point is, while this discomfort is rooted, in part, in the content of messages (the impossibility of the ideal), it reflects the historically specific relationship between women and their bodies, which is rooted in a more general reification of the social world.

CONCLUSION: INTERVENTION AS MATERIAL CHANGE

However valid the observation that the context of eating disorders is one of distorted imagery of women, this approach cannot explain the specific rather than general patterns of the disease. While the major contribution of feminist analyses has been to link anorexia to issues of power or patriarchal relations, relations of class have not been explored. This paper is an attempt to raise and partly answer questions about the link between anorexia and class structure, between patriarchal and class relations. In order to do so, we must reject the view of consciousness as simply reflecting or internalizing cultural values as one-sided. From the insights of de Beauvoir in particular, we should explore the development of consciousness of self in relationship to the material conditions of women's existence. Consciousness occurs dialectically through both the externalization of oneself through our day-to-day activities – or labour – and the internalization of cultural meanings assigned to those activities. This requires that we examine women's interactive relationship to both the material and nonmaterial dimensions of social existence. At the level of individual experience, class places women in a particular relationship to the benefits of women's liberation. Reflecting the contradictory nature of this liberation, adolescent women from professional success-oriented families receive contradictory double messages about their identity as women: while the rhetoric of women's liberation rewards girls for nontraditional aspirations and achievements, processes operate at the material level to undermine women's real autonomy. In other words, women are encouraged to think about themselves as autonomous Subjects, while the demands associated with divisions of labour in both the labour force and the family give priority to women's lives as wives and mothers. There is conflict between consciousness of self as being "for-self" and being "for-others." Without material changes in the existential conditions of women's existence, the wider the spread of rhetoric and imagery of women's liberation, the more generalized this conflict is apt to be.

At the general level, class is linked to the historically specific relationship between consciousness of self and body. In advanced capitalist societies, this relationship is gender specific. This brief paper identifies three interrelated processes whereby this relationship is constructed as the historical and material precondition of anorexia: the linking of women's future to men through roles which perpetuate their status as being for-others; the cultivation of a general anxiety about the body as affirmation of femininity and, hence, of male approval; the separation of body as an object of transformation and self as a specific form of more generalized reified consciousness. From this perspective, more than cultural change is required. The elimination of eating disorders requires change at the material level. The point is not that women individually relearn a more appropriate assessment of their body image or their relationship to food – as Fonda suggests – but that women's relationship to their bodies be transformed. At the individual level, this requires development of self as an intellectual rather than merely physical presence through self-affirming activity. At the collective level, this links the struggles for women's mental health to those for the transformation of the conditions of existence for both men and women.

NOTES

1 While this describes the epidemiology of anorexia until very recently, Garfinkel and Garner (1982) report that current diagnoses increasingly include older women, women from working-class familes, and men. Although these categories remain a distinct minority, this suggests the democratization of eating disorders – a discussion beyond the scope of this paper but accounted for by the type of explanation sketched below.

2 For problems of estimating the frequency of eating disorders, see Currie (1988).

3 Orbach argues that a girl first learns about her social role through the mother – daughter relationship. Within this relationship the girl becomes exposed to her mother's own ambivalence about motherhood. Specifically, the mother must teach the daughter the strictures of patriarchy: defer to others; anticipate and meet the needs of others; seek self-definition through connection with others. Added to this are two taboos for women: they must not express the need to be nurtured and they must not initiate. Thus the mother will simultaneously reject the daughter's dependency as well as her desire for autonomy. The result is that the mother prevents the daughter's psychological separation. The ensuing insecurity reemerges during adolescence, when it is shifted to an insecurity in relation to one's body. As others have noted, this analysis fosters "mother-blame."

4 Johnson argues that those suffering from bulimia were born in the 1960s and grew up in a time of shifting cultural norms *caused* by the feminist movement (emphasis mine). To support this he notes that there has been growing pressure on women to achieve and yet no clear way for them to live up to these expectations of achievement (*Leader Post*, 12 November 1986).

5 While de Beauvoir's existentialism is a critique of classical idealism, a number of problems make the wholesale acceptance of this approach unsuitable. Serious limitations include her uncritical acceptance of masculinity and masculine ways of acting in the world as appropriate goals for women; her view of human relations as inherently conflictual; the failure to explain power differences between men and women as social because they are treated *a priori*; the universalization of the terms "man" and "woman." She herself dismisses historical materialism as useful, citing in particular the work of Engels. Nonetheless, the observations which follow are an extension of her view of women as the "Second Sex," and the failure to acknowledge this influence would represent a serious error.

6 A number of researchers claim that nontraditional aspirations in women are perceived by many men as threatening. In a study of mate selection, for example, Center (1975) correctly hypothesized that unless a man is particularly secure, he is likely to find achievement in a future partner threatening.

7 It is perhaps salient to note here that Jane Fonda, an advocate of physical fitness programs, herself suffered from bulimia for twenty-three years (*Leader Post* 1984).

8 *See* "The Man With the Golden Scalpel: Repairing the Ravages of Time" in *Maclean's*, June 1975.

9 It has been estimated that 56 per cent of American women between the ages of 24 and 54 are dieters (Schwartz, Thompson, and Johnson 1985). While there seems to be no similar polls of Canadian women, an unpublished survey of grade 10 and 12 female students in a Saskatoon high school reveals that, by Grade 12, 76 per cent of schoolgirls report that they diet, 12 per cent use dieting aids, 17 per cent use vomiting, and 7 per cent use purgatives to assist in weight loss (discussed in Currie 1988).

REFERENCES

Advisory Council on the Status of Women 1985. *Women and Work*, Ottawa: Advisory Council on the Status of Women.

Baker, M. 1985. *What Will Tomorrow Bring? ... A study of the aspirations of Adolescent Women*. Ottawa: Advisory Council on the Status of Women.

Bennett W.B. and J. Gurin 1982. *The Dieter's Dilemma: Eating Less and Weighing More*. New York: Basic Books.

Bersheid, E. and E. Walster 1974. "Physical Attractiveness." In R. Berowitz, ed., *Advances in Experimental Social Psychology*. New York: Academic Press.

Boskind-White, M. 1985. "Bulimia: A Sociocultural Perspective." In S.W. Emmett, ed., *Theory and Treatment of Anorexia Nervosa and Bulimia.* New York: Brunner/Mazel.

"Bulemia Linked to Feminism." *Leader Post,* 12 November 1986.

Chernin, K. 1982. *The Obsession: Reflections on the Tyranny of Slenderness.* New York: Harper and Row.

Cottin-Pogrebin, L. 1983. "The Power of Beauty." *Ms.* (December issue).

Center, R. 1975. *Sexual Attractiveness and Love: An Instrument Theory.* Springfield, Illinois: C.C. Thomas.

Currie, D.H. 1988. "Starvation Amidst Abundance: Female Adolescents and Anorexia." In B.S. Bolaria and H. Dickinson, eds., *Sociology of Health Care in Canada.* Toronto: Harcourt, Brace, Jovanovich.

de Beauvoir, S. 1952. *The Second Sex.* New York: Bantam Books.

"Eating Disorders Increase Sixfold." *Globe and Mail* (Toronto) 27 October 1986.

"Eating Problem Poses Danger." *Leader Post,* 31 December 1984.

Garfinkel, P.E. and D.M. Garner 1982. *Anorexia Nervosa: A Multidimensional Perspective.* New York: Brunner/Mazel.

Gault, J. 1975. "The Man With the Golden Scalpel: Repairing the Ravages of Time." *Maclean's* (June issue).

Goffman, E. 1976. *Gender Advertisement.* New York: Harper Colophon.

Greer, G. 1970. *The Female Eunuch.* London: Granada.

Leonard, D. 1980. *Sex and Generation: A Study of Courtship and Weddings.* London: Tavistock.

Orbach, S. 1978. *Fat is a Feminist Issue.* New York: Paddington.

Orbach, S. 1986. *Hunger Strike: An Anorexic's Struggle as a Metaphor for Our Age.* New York: W.W. Norton.

Ortner, S.B. 1972. "Is Female to Male as Nature Is to Culture?" *Feminist Studies* 1(2): 5–31.

Richmond-Abbott, M. 1983. *Masculine and Feminine: Sex Roles Over the Life Cycle.* New York: Random House.

Sartre, J.P. 1969. *Being and Nothingness.* New York: Washington Square.

Schwartz, D.M., M.G. Thompson, and C.L. Johnson 1985. "Anorexia Nervosa and Bulimia: The Sociocultural Context." In S.W. Emmett, ed., *Theory and Treatment of Anorexia Nervosa and Bulimia.* New York: Brunner/Mazel.

Sutherland, S. 1978. "The Ambitious Female: Women's Low Professional Aspirations" *Signs* 3: 774–94.

Szekely, E.A. 1987a. "Cinderella's Stepsisters Revisited: The Problem of the Body." Unpublished paper, Department of Sociology in Education, Ontario Institute for Studies in Education.

Szekely, E.A. 1987b. "Society, Ideology, and the Relentless Pursuit of Thinness." *Practice: The Journal of Politics, Economics, Psychology, Sociology and Culture* 3.

Szekely, E.A. 1987c. "Women's Anxious Pursuit of Attractive Appearance."
   Phenomenology and Pedagogy 5(2): 108–18.
Thompson, M.G. and M.T. Gans 1985. "Do Anorexics and Bulimics Get
   Well? In S.W. Emmett, ed., *Theory and Treatment of Anorexia and Bulimia*.
   New York: Brunner/Mazel.

DORIS MᶜILROY

Towards an Understanding of the Social Logic Underlying Women's Sporting Practices

In this chapter, Doris McIlroy examines the sporting tastes of two groups of Canadian women occupying positions remote from each other in social space. They are identified as manual workers, with low economic and cultural capital, and professional women in the visual arts, with relatively high economic and cultural capital. The theoretical insights and concepts of the French sociologist Pierre Bourdieu were used to help us grasp the specific social logic (at times, an unconscious social logic) underlying the sporting tastes and distastes of the two social groups. A certain systematic ordering of sporting tastes was visible, and an analysis of these tastes suggested that the distribution of sporting preferences and practices was related to a disposition toward the body conditioned by volume and composition of capital.

Vers une compréhension de la logique sociale sous-tendant les activités sportives des femmes

Cet article examine les goûts en matière de sports de deux groupes de Canadiennes se trouvant dans des positions éloignées l'un de l'autre dans la hiérarchie sociale. Il s'agit d'une part de travailleuses manuelles, dont le capital économique et culturel est faible, et d'autre part de professionnelles du domaine des arts visuels jouissant d'un capital économique et culturel relativement élevé. En utilisant des concepts et des intuitions théoriques du sociologue français Pierre Bourdieu, l'auteure tente de saisir la logique sociale spécifique – et parfois inconsciente sous-tendant les préférences et les aversions des deux groupes en matière de sports. Les résultats ont révélé une certaine classification systématique des préférences en matière de sports en fonction de la classe sociale, et une analyse de ces résultats laisse supposer que la répartition des préférences et des habitudes dans ce domaine était reliée à une disposition à l'endroit du corps dépendant de l'importance et de la composition du capital.

In the past, the study of social phenomena has tended to be empirically based, primarily focused on isolating causal factors. My research takes a different approach. I have attempted to take into account the causal power of structures operating independently of the consciousness of agents in order to have a deeper understanding of social reality. I tried to think the social world in a relational way rather than in a linear way in keeping with the theoretical framework developed by the French sociologist, Pierre Bourdieu.

Bourdieu has developed a theoretical frame of reference which allows us to include symbolic capital and power as well as economic capital and power in our analysis. Some of his concepts (for example, social space, class habitus, relation to one's own body, or cultural capital) may be unfamiliar to some. But if we are to use his theoretical insights and logic to help us understand and explain social reality, it is imperative that we also use his concepts.

The aim of this study is to try to grasp the specific social logic underlying the sporting tastes and distastes of two groups of women occupying positions remote from each other in social space and living in an androcentric culture. Do their sporting preferences and practices follow some sort of pattern or are they a random assortment of tastes? If some pattern is visible, what is the specific social logic which might account for this systematic ordering?

Before examining some of the sporting practices and perceptions of practices of the two social groups, we should briefly review Bourdieu's theoretical position in order to "set the stage," so to speak, and familiarize the reader with some of his basic concepts.

BOURDIEU'S THEORETICAL POSITION

Bourdieu's theoretical framework[1] is a valuable conceptual tool for investigating social phenomena since it allows one to escape from an ordinary acceptance of the social order. In the past, social research has tended to reduce the scientific order to androcentric perceptions of the social order; the structures of power which condition such perceptions are rarely taken into account. Bourdieu's theory goes beyond understanding the social world from an androcentric or gyocentric perspective, but rather takes into account structures of thought – that is, visions of the social world which themselves contribute to the construction of this world – and also the structures of power which condition such visions or perceptions. In the words of Brubaker (1985, 747), "he constructs a general theory of the 'economy of symbolic goods' and its relation to the material economy –

a theory of the production and consumption of symbolic goods, the pursuit of symbolic capital, and the modes of conversion of symbolic capital or power into other forms of power."

Rather than conceptualizing an explanatory model of social reality in oppositions of subjectivity – objectivity, Bourdieu's theory goes further; it attempts to unite in a scientific method these two ways of understanding the social world. On one side, it allows for reflexive, subjective expressions of experiences of the social world, and on the other, it takes into account the objective structures conditioning these expressions (Bourdieu 1987, 148–50).

Bourdieu employs the concepts "habitus" and "class habitus" as primary tools of scientific discourse to characterize the mediating structure between conditions of existence and practices. This mediating structure he visualizes as internalized, incorporated, embodied social structures. He defines class habitus as "the internalized form of class condition and of the conditionings it entails" (Bourdieu 1984, 101). Other authors (for example, Hegel, Weber, Durkheim, and Mauss) have also used the concept habitus. For Mauss (1950, 369), the word "habitus" includes the triple point of view of the person, that is, the biological, social, and psychological person. What Mauss expresses as the triple point of view of the whole person, Bourdieu calls the unity of the subjective conscience. "The habitus is both the generative principle of objectively classifiable judgements and the system of classification ... of these practices" (Bourdieu, 1984, 170). Bourdieu's use of the term "habitus" as synonymous with "system of dispositions" expresses the transformation of experiences of social structures into intrinsic, coherent, unconscious social logics. "Relation to one's own body" is another key concept used by Bourdieu. This he sees as a fundamental aspect of the habitus, or privileged dimension of the habitus, since it is through the body that each class enacts its practical philosophy (Bourdieu 1984, 190–94).

THE STUDY

In this study, women are seen as active agents in the construction of culture, active agents in society. The choices they make are sometimes choices of necessity, reflecting material conditions of existence, gender conditions of existence, age, or social trajectory, but choices none the less.

Women representing extreme positions in social space – that is, those with low economic and cultural capital and those with relatively high economic and cultural capital, were interviewed. The former are identified as manual workers and the latter as artistic producers.

These women (six in one group and seven in the other) were Canadians (that is, born in Canada or having lived in Canada at least twenty years), living in Ottawa, between the ages of thirty and fifty, working in the paid labour force, and having at least one child. The manual workers were represented by full-time workers at McDonalds, cleaners, and a factory worker; the artistic producers were university professors in the visual arts and museum and art gallery curators and administrators.

The central focus of this study is one's relation to the body, which Bourdieu called "a fundamental aspect of the habitus which distinguishes the working classes from the privileged classes" (Bourdieu 1978, 838). According to Bourdieu, "the logic whereby agents incline towards this or that sporting practice cannot be understood unless their dispositions towards sport, which are themselves one dimension of a particular relation to the body, are reinserted into the unity of the system of dispositions, the habitus, which is the basis from which life-styles are generated" (Bourdieu 1978, 833).

Tables 1 and 2 show regular and non-regular sporting practices the two groups. Bowling, walking, and baseball were regular practices of the manual workers, whereas the artistic producers were active in exercise classes, tennis, walking, and swimming. Both groups also participated in non-regular sporting practices; waterskiing, skidooing, and camping were favoured by the manual workers and crosscountry skiing and cycling by the artistic producers. Tennis, canoeing, and crosscountry skiing were practices common to both groups, but with a difference, the difference being the modality of practices.

In attempting to understand the meaning sport holds for each group, as well as the expected benefits and profits, differences in modality need to be taken into account along with differences in practices. For the manual worker, walking consisted of walking a small dog around the block, whereas several of the artistic producers walked to and from work, approximately two to three miles per day. The artistic producers belonged to tennis clubs, whereas for the manual worker, tennis was a make-up game against the side of the school. In crosscountry skiing, the manual workers skied on flat easy trails unlike the artistic producers, who liked to work up a sweat in the Gatineau Hills. In general, the mode of physical activity preferred by the professional group was one which required considerable physical effort, whereas the manual workers were inclined toward easier practices. However, the manual workers liked the speed and excitement of going fast, but a speed generated outside the body.

Table 1
Regular Sporting Practices of Manual Workers and Professionals

Group	Physical activity
Manual Workers	
McDonalds 1	No regular physical activity
McDonalds 2	Walks dog every day, approximately 1 km
McDonalds 3	Baseball team at husband's work in summer
School cleaner	No regular physical activity
Molly Maid	No regular physical activity
Factory worker	Weekly bowling
Professionals	
AP 1	Heart condition; formerly very active (tennis twice per week; exercised every day)
AP 2	Exercise class two noon hours per week; swimming three times per week during pregnancy
AP 3	Aerobics three times per week; weight lifting two times per week; walks approximately one hour per day
AP 4	Exercise class once a week
AP 5	Pre- and postnatal exercises; used to jog and lift weights
AP 6	Walks one hour per day; used to jog and lift weights before child was born
AP 7	Swimming once per week; used to exercise every day and walk to work; now has no time

TASTES AND DISTASTES OF EACH GROUP

Along with data concerning their regular and non-regular sporting practices, information concerning practices that do or do not appeal was also solicited. Table 3 summarizes the tastes and distastes of each group.

With few exceptions, the tastes of the manual workers were the distastes of the artistic producers. Curling and bodybuilding (building muscle bulk) were two exceptions; neither group found these appealing. These similarities will be discussed briefly, but the primary concern of this paper is to look at some of the differences and work backwards attempting to get a glimpse of the social logic behind these differences.

Similarities

Both groups rejected curling, but for different reasons. The artistic producers, it seems, reject curling for the same reason they reject bowling, because of the social composition of the individuals who participate in these sports. Some openly expressed their rejections

Table 2
Non-regular Sporting Practices of Manual Workers and Professionals

Group	Physical Activity
Manual Workers	
McDonalds 1	Camping, pool, dancercise class once after pregnancy
McDonalds 2	Waterskiing, tennis against wall, fishing, crosscountry skiing on flat trails
McDonalds 3	Waterskiing, camping, fishing, skidooing
School Cleaner	Skidooing, snow shovelling, camping, biking, lying out in the sun
Molly Maid	Skating, biking to the pool, swimming, canoeing
Factory worker	Skidooing, walking, horseshoes, biking, sandbags boating, dancercise class once after surgery
Professionals	
AP 1	Skating, swimming, cycling, class crosscountry skiing in Gatineau Hills
AP 2	Crosscountry skiing in Gatineau Hills
AP 3	Cycling, swimming, crosscountry skiing
AP 4	Biking, swimming, crosscountry skiing, walking dog
AP 5	Crosscountry skiing, farm chores
AP 6	Skating, playing with children
AP 7	Biking and canoeing

in terms of class distinction, whereas others were more subtle. Rejections reflect a sense of place, that is, a feeling of not fitting in. They sense they would not fit in because the people they might meet there are not people like themselves: "That's totally alien to my experience, I think that's a rural game" (artist-curator 3); "I was a championship curler as a high school student, but I wouldn't do it now to save my life ... It is the same as bowling, so inside and noisy" (artist-professor 5). The manual workers say it is boring and too slow. "It's boring, it doesn't look all that exciting – sweeping that ball around" (Molly Maid); "I think it is too much work – fighting with this broom" (factory worker). They enjoyed team sports such as bowling or baseball, but curling was classed as boring work.

The artistic producers reject curling for the same reason they reject bowling; it brings no distinctions. Like curling, "bowling is, excuse the expression just sort of half-assed, I mean it is not really a sport to me" (artist-professor 6); "The people I know associate bowling as a sort of lower middle class thing – there's a class distinction" (artist-professor 5). Embedded in these comments associating curling with bowling is the notion that these sports bring no distinctions. Bowling is considered vulgar, that is, "half-assed," and "not even a sport"; although views about curling were not expressed

Table 3
Sporting Tastes of Each Social Group

Group	Likes	Dislikes
Manual workers	Bowling	Curling
	Snowmobiling	Fencing
	Western riding	Sailing
	Judo and karate	Bodybuilding
	Camping	
	Waterskiing	
	Fishing	
	Swimming	
Professionals	Fencing	Bowling
	Riding	Curling
	Sailing	Wrestling
	Exercises classes	Bodybuilding
	Tennis	Judo and karate
	Crosscountry skiing	Snowmobiling; all types of
	Walking	racing vehicles (dirt bikes,
	Jogging	racing boats, motorcycling,
	Biking	racing cars)

in such explicit terms, nevertheless, the association is unmistakable. Therefore, it seems fair to say that the rejection of curling by the artistic producers seems to be associated with the notion that it brings no distinctions and that it is alien to their urban experiences.

Although all the manual workers rejected curling, the rationale behind rejections was not completely clear. Perhaps it is associated with the mystery around sweeping the stone, since several remarked on the sweeping. Team sports like bowling and baseball may be favoured because they are more commonplace and less formal. They can muster the economic and cultural capital for bowling but curling demands more. One must have the skills or at least know people who curl in order to make up a team, and the technique is a little more specialized. So it seems that a logic of necessity governs the manual workers' rejection of curling, whereas, the artistic producers' rejections appear to be based on a logic of distinction.

As might be expected, hockey and football were ignored by both groups. This might be explained as a result of their gender conditions of existence. Bodybuilding (that is, building muscle bulk) was also rejected by both groups mainly because it goes against female canons of beauty. It is interesting to note, however, that the manual workers phrase their rejections in terms of appropriateness whereas the artistic producers speak in terms of what is aesthetically pleasing.

"This muscle stuff is ridiculous, that's not a woman, that's blaaah – I mean that's for men" (school cleaner); "It is esthetically unappealing, I don't like those big muscled figures; in fact I find it revolting" (artist-administrator 4). The manual workers seem to express their disposition toward the body in a realistic, pragmatic way, concentrating on substance or content rather than form, and the artistic producers seem to show an aesthetic disposition, focusing on form rather than content. This will become more evident as other expressions of their perceptions and appreciations are presented.

Differences

Three outstanding differences were as follows:

- The artistic producers participated regularly in exercise classes while the manual workers did not.

- The manual workers exhibited a taste for motorized sports whereas the artistic producers had a profound distaste for these activities.

- The manual workers rejected sailing and fencing and the artistic producers found these sports appealing.

Exercise Classes

One of the outstanding differences between the groups is the fact that the artistic producers regularly attend exercise classes and the manual workers do not. Economic concerns alone cannot account for this difference, since camping gear and waterskiing equipment (two sports popular with the manual workers) also require considerable economic investment. In reality, if money can be found for these activities, it could be used instead for exercise classes. Why do the manual workers choose to invest time, energy, and money in waterskiing rather than exercise class? One answer might be that, for manual workers, the profits from exercise classes do not match the investment. Unlike the artistic producers, they do not gain a professional profit. A trim, slim figure increases the artistic producers' chances of professional advancement, but the manual workers can expect no such return.

The expense of exercise classes might be the reason offered for not participating, but on closer inspection we may see other reasons. Boltanski (1971, 217) found that, in France, the interest and attention individuals give their bodies were not the same for all social groups. His analysis showed that attention to health matters, indicated by one's attention to preventive medicine, grows as one moves from the working class to the professional class. The comments of the artistic producers in this study seem to echo these findings; none smoked, and they appeared to be more concerned with their weight and their health in general than the manual workers. The fact that they knew exactly what they weighed before they were pregnant or five years ago suggests they paid close attention to their weight. Artist-professor 6 summed up the situation for the entire group when she said, "I think I have a sort of body image which is a quite thin ideal body image."

The manual workers, while not wishing to be obese, seemed to tolerate more fat on their bodies. When asked if they ever tried to lose weight, the manual workers replied: "I should, but I don't" (Molly Maid); "I figure if you get to a certain weight, you have always been that weight, why change something ... because half the time you look sick after you lose weight" (McDonald worker 2); "If I lose it, I lose it, if I don't, I don't, as long as I don't gain too much" (school cleaner). So it seems the manual workers appear more content with their bodies; they also said their mates preferred women with a little "meat on them"; therefore they see little profit in trying to make themselves slimmer.

Artist-curator 3 goes to aerobic and weightlifting classes for health reasons. "I'm forty ... I've seen my body change already and I want to forestall change as much as I can ... I do it primarily for health and looks, which I think in this respect are connected." Artist-curator 2 says, "My husband and I crosscountry skied a lot ... but the only formal thing I do is an exercise class – I love it – I'd like to do it more. I feel it is my time. It is not just for my body it is for my head ... I think it is extremely important for mental as well as physical health."

These comments and feelings about exercise classes or slimming practices give some glimpse of the different dispositions toward the body of each social group. For the manual workers, the maintenance of a slim body was nor part of their disposition toward the body, not part of their class habitus. For them, the profits from exercise classes do not match their investment of time, money, and energy. The artistic producers, however, expect a physical profit – that is, a fit and healthy body, an indirect socio-professional profit (part of being a professional is the professional look) and a personal profit – time for oneself.

Motorized Sports

The artistic producers expressed a vehement dislike for all motorized sports – dirt bikes, motorboats, motorcycling and car racing, all of which are sports which appeal to the manual workers. "I love watching car racing, or boat racing ... Two of them just touching! Holy cow! Some of them wipe out real well ... I love snowmobiling, just racing across the snow, like, I love the outdoors" (school cleaner). "Up at the camp, my parents have a rowboat with a motor on it ... and in the winter we go skidooing" (factory worker). "Waterskiing is fun ... It's fast, but you don't really notice it" (McDonalds worker 3). These sports, apprehended through schemes of perception and appreciation of their class habitus, are compatible with the disposition the manual workers have toward the body. That is to say, focusing on substance or content, they seem to appreciate the fun, the speed and excitement of movement, and the element of risk and danger.

The artistic producers detest snowmobiling. "I think snowmobiling is – polluting the landscape, you know, with noise ... It is ugly to me – why can't people go in a sailboat as opposed to a speedboat?" (artist-professor 6). "I hate it, and I think it is offensive to everyone around. I love going through the countryside on crosscountry skis, but these hooligans, I mean that's really the way they impress you ... It is the same thing with noisy boats, I really think it is unnecessary" (artist-administrator 4). "I can't bear the noise of them ... They are so intrusive, they can go anywhere, and one other thing I like about winter is that suddenly nature doesn't allow you to go everywhere, and if you do, you go in quietly on skis – sort of much more as a part of nature. The idea of zooming through it is just totally repulsive to me" (artist-professor 5).

The intolerances expressed by the artistic producers objectifies their sense of distinction. Consciously or unconsciously, they appear to seek to separate themselves from the common lot. They see, through their schemes of perception and appreciation, these activities as desecrating nature, a profanity, as opposed to crosscountry skiing, which is viewed as an activity which allows one to honour or worship nature away from the hordes of noisy, crass people, "the hooligans," in select places – silent, clean and lofty.

These statements also objectify their relation to the body. They object to the noise; it pollutes their environment and it pollutes their ears. They see no profit in these sports; they prefer sports like sailing or crosscountry skiing, sports which require an investment of knowledge, skill, or bodily training. This was particularly evident in their comments about sailing and fencing.

Fencing and Sailing

Perceptions and appreciations of fencing and sailing were found to be markedly different for the two groups. Concerning fencing, the artistic producers offered the following remarks: "I've done fencing when I was younger, I think it is very artistic. It is a very good workout too" (artist-curator 1). "I did it one year at university, I think it is very graceful" (artist-administrator 4). "It seems very graceful, I like the tensions that the bodies go through ... psychologically very interesting between the two fences" (artist-curator 7). "It appeals more than other things, again because of the agility required and the thinking, and I guess the sort of dancelike quality of it" (artist-professor 5).

The manual workers show a different dispostion. "Oh no, I don't like that, that's violent, I'd be too afraid of getting the end of it" (factory worker). "It just doesn't make much sense to me, I've never met anyone in my life who did that" (McDonald worker 1). "I've never had any desire to fence, maybe because it seems violent" (McDonald worker 3).

On one side are found perceptions and appreciations through which qualities of the body such as agility, strength, tension, and intellectuality are admired, while on the other side perceptions and social judgements of fencing were identified with violence. The former have their origins in an ascetic aesthetic disposition toward the body and the latter in a pragmatic, realistic disposition toward the body.

The manual workers, expressing a realistic disposition toward the body, centre their attention on the content of the activity, the actual actions of two bodies slicing and poking at each other with long sharp knives. Given their schemes of perception and appreciation it seems only logical they might find it distasteful. The artistic producers, following the schemes of perception and appreciation of an aesthetic, ascetic dispostion toward the body, concern themselves with the art form of movement. They seem to ignore the actual mechanics of the physical happening and see rather the "dancelike quality" or the "tension of the bodies." It seems quite sensible, quite logical, given their schemes of perception and appreciation, that they find fencing elegant and artistic.

The rationale underlying the manual worker's distaste for sailing appears more subtle. "No, I don't like sailing at all" (factory worker). "Nay – that's too slow. Give me a power boat and you're talking fun" (school cleaner). "No, but going on a yacht cruise would [appeal to me]. I don't know anybody that sails" (McDonalds worker 1). The fact that the manual workers oppose waterskiing to sailing, or find it too slow may be seen as a subtle expression of their relation to the body. They do not see any fun in sailing: "that's too slow"; fun is going fast. Also, their friends do not sail, so they may be seen as feeling "out of place" in the sailing milieu.

Like fencing or crosscountry skiing, sailing sets one apart; it is a sign of mastery, a sign of distinction. "I like the fact that there is no noise except for the wind. I love the chance – you are dependent on the wind to propel you, and the skill of finding the wind and bringing the boat around. I like the skill ... you don't pollute and you don't make noise" (artist-curator 2).

Poceille (1981, 190–3) found that the privileged class tend to make an art form of sport. He says that those with high cultural capital take information and knowledge, combine it with mastering equilibrium and other features of the body, and match these with natural elements, wind, sun, or snow, to get the maximum effect from a light, simple machine. Because of their high economic and cultural capital, the privileged class can invest knowledge and training in the development of bodily skills such as those used in fencing and sailing. These sports are emblems of distinction signifying distance from necessity.

CONCLUSION

Based on the information supplied by the two social groups, it appears that bodily practices, and sporting practices in particular, were not the result of a random series of choices and rejections but rather seem to be structured in a coherent manner. A relationship of affinity appeared to exist in the sporting tastes of individuals from the same social group, while a relationship of opposition was visible between groups, except when gender conditionings were a pertinent factor. The evidence seems to suggest that the distribution of sporting tastes between the two social groups was governed by a system of dispositions conditioned by structures related to the social division of labour and the sexual division of labour.

NOTES

1 For a thorough understanding of Bourdieu's theoretical position, see his *Distinction: A Social Analysis of the Judgement of Taste* (1984) and *Choses dites* (1987).

BIBLIOGRAPHY

Boltanski, L. 1971. "Les usages sociaux du corps." *Annales Economics-sociétés-civilisations* 1: 195–233.

Bourdieu, P. 1968. "Structuralism and Theory of Sociological Knowledge." *Social Research* 35(4): 681–706.

Bourdieu, P. 1977a. *Outline of a Theory of Practice*. Cambridge, England: Cambridge University Press.

Bourdieu, P. 1977b. "Remarques provisoires sur la perception sociale du corps." *Actes de la recherche en sciences sociales*. 14: 31–34.

Bourdieu, P. 1977c. "Symbolic power." Tr. C. Wringe. In D. Gleeson, ed., *Identity and Structure: Issues in the Sociology of Education*. Nafferton, England: Nafferton Books.

Bourdieu, P. 1978. "Sport and Social Class." *Social Science Information* 17(6): 819–40.

Bourdieu, P. 1980. *Le sens pratique*. Paris: Les Éditions de Minuit.

Bourdieu, P. 1984. *Distinction: A Social Critique of the Judgement of Taste*. Tr. R. Nice. Cambridge, Mass.: Harvard University Press.

Bourdieu, P. 1987. *Choses dites*. Paris: Les Éditions de Minuit.

Brubaker, R. 1985. "Rethinking Classical Theory." *Theory and Society* 14: 745–75.

Mauss, M. 1950. "Notion de technique du corps." In M. Mauss, ed., *Sociologie et anthropologie*. Paris: Presses Universitaires de France.

Poceille, C. 1979. "Pratiques sportives et demandes sociales." *Travaux et recherches en Éducation physique et sportive*. Institut Supérieur d'Éducation Permanente 5:31–48.

MEGAN BARKER DAVIES

The Women beyond the Gates: Female Mental Health Patients in British Columbia, 1910–1935[1]

This article considers the experience of female patients who entered British Columbia's mental health institutions between 1910 and 1935. For these women, life in the asylum community was shaped by institutional routine, patients' labour, and rigid gender divisions. Yet within this ordered sphere, women sought to recreate elements of the female culture they had left behind through the relationships they formed and the kinds of resistance they used to express their dissatisfaction.

Les femmes au-delà des barrières
Les patientes des hôpitaux psychiatriques en Colombie-Britannique,
1910–1935

Cet article traite de l'expérience des patientes admises dans les hôpitaux psychiatriques en Colombie-Britannique entre 1910 et 1935. Pour ces femmes, la vie à l'asile était marquée par la routine institutionnelle, les tâches à effectuer et la ségrégation. Pourtant, au sein de cette organisation, les femmes essayaient de recréer des éléments de la culture féminine qu'elle avaient laissée derrière elles par l'entremise des relations qu'elles établissaient et des formes de résistance qu'elles utilisaient pour exprimer leur insatisfaction.

INTRODUCTION

We know little about women who were patients in Canada's mental health institutions in the early twentieth century. While a body of literature is developing about the nineteenth century mental health field in Canada, and although feminist scholars have analyzed the gender dynamics of our contemporary mental health care system,

only a few scholars have considered gender in the historical material
(Mitchinson 1987, McLaren 1986, Shortt 1986). Nonetheless, as our
knowledge of structures and patterns becomes more complete, the
asylum gates are beginning to swing open.

In an effort to understand the experience of female mental health
patients in early twentieth-century Canada, this paper will focus on
the institutional experience of women who entered British Columbia's mental health facilities between 1910 and 1935. I will explore
the boundaries and structures which the asylum imposed on the
patients and consider how women were able to personalize the institutional world of the asylum. Using the concept of female culture
and examining the gender-specific ways in which women responded
to institutionalization, I shall look at the asylum experience as it was
defined both by the institution and by the women who entered as
patients (Conrad 1984, Lebsock 1984). We find that the experiences
of women as patients were shaped by the character of institutional
life itself and by the contours of female culture.[2] This paper is an
exploration of these themes, a conversation with the women who
stand just beyond the asylum gates, waiting for us to listen.[3]

INSTITUTIONAL LIFE

British Columbia's first provincial asylum was established in Victoria
in 1872. In 1878, with a total of thirty-seven patients, the asylum
moved to New Westminster, a settlement not far from Vancouver.
In 1913, a second mental health institution, Essondale, was built not
far from the older New Westminster asylum. The growth of the two
institutions between 1910 and 1935 was dynamic: one small institution, housing 595 patients, was transformed by 1935 into two complexes which held a total of 2,823 patients.[4] Of the 595 people who
were confined in New Westminster in 1910, 28.8 per cent were
women. By the end of the period this figure increased to 35.6
per cent.[5]

The institutional structures of the New Westminster and Essondale
asylums impinged on the lives of women who entered them as patients in a number of ways. Because of the growing numbers of
patients, the asylum was often overcrowded and impersonal. However, the administration sought to organize the lives of patients
through admission procedures, daily routine, and patient labour.
Consequently, patient life was rigidly gender-defined.

When we look more carefully at the patient populations of the
two institutions we find that male and female patients were not
equally dispersed between New Westminster and Essondale. Statis-

tical information drawn from the annual reports shows that, from the completion of Essondale in 1913 until 1930, when the female chronic building at Essondale was finally ready for occupation, New Westminster was primarily occupied by women and Essondale by men. Although the gender separation between the two institutions was not complete, it did, in effect, create two separate spaces – one male and one female. Female patients at New Westminster lived in what was primarily a female world, their contact with men limited to physicians, male staff, and the occasional visitor.

Larger numbers of patients meant that both institutions suffered from chronic overcrowding. Notwithstanding the opening of Essondale in 1913, annual reports of the period, particularly during the 1920s and 1930s, indicate that living conditions within the asylums were crowded (Annual Report 1925, R14). In 1928 the medical superintendent, Dr A.L. Crease, noted that the female side of the institution was particularly overcrowded, adding that he was looking forward to the completion of the new female chronic building (Annual Report 1928, X10). And by 1934 Crease was warning that overcrowded conditions increased the number of acute and chronic cases and created a potentially dangerous environment in New Westminster's older non-fireproofed buildings (Annual Report 1934, Q10–11).

The growing numbers of patients confined in New Westminster and Essondale also meant that routine and organization were increasingly crucial to the smooth functioning of the institution[6] (Francis 1981, 7). Consequently, the daily lives of women inside the two institutions were circumscribed of institutional codes, implicit and explicit, that related specifically to the internal workings of the asylum community. Daily routine, while clearly a necessary part of a functional institution, probably served to nullify the stated purpose of the institution – the treatment of the mentally ill (Lasch 1973, 7). Furthermore, asylum routine was as much a means of establishing the authority of the staff as it was a policy of effective and efficient asylum management.

Initiation into asylum routine began when a woman first entered the asylum. Personal items such as jewelry and letters that the patient had brought with her were catalogued and put away; a patient number was assigned; the patient was examined for any bruises or markings, thus absolving the asylum of responsibility for injuries acquired prior to committal. Patients were also given institutional clothing. The women, the superintendent reported were, "dressed in plain, serviceable, one-piece gingham dresses and also ... fully clothed in respect to underclothing" (Provincial Secretary's Correspondence,

Box 13, File 5). In the last step of the admission process, the patient was bathed and put to bed under observation. A quiet, cooperative patient, like Mrs. W in 1920, would be "allowed up on the ward" the same day she arrived, while other more disruptive patients might remain in bed for their first week at the asylum[7] (Patient no. 6465). This admission routine, which remained unaltered throughout the period, served to begin the institutionalization of patients by taking away individual personal belongings and establishing the authority of staff and physicians.

The case histories allow us glimpse into how female patients felt when they were first thrust into the institution. Gerald Grob argues that admission to a mental hospital of this period would have been a frightening experience (Grob 1983, 15). Certainly, a sense of disorientation is strongly suggested by several of the case histories. An elderly woman, Mrs. P, told the asylum doctor after her admission that "it [the asylum] is all so strange to her" (Patient no. 11051). For some women the asylum would eventually become a place that approximated home, but many continued to express their dissatisfaction with the asylum. Five months after her admission, it was reported that Mrs. P "mixes agreeably with her associates," yet she never stopped asking for her release.

Women who entered the asylum as patients likely found the asylum a clamorous, busy, and rather confusing place. Certainly many patients were noisy. Mrs. S, for instance, sang constantly throughout the day for several months (Patient no. 6330). The loudness of the asylum prompted Miss J, a young woman, to write a letter to one of the asylum doctors, telling him that "this afternoon my nerves were all on edge, and for the racket that was going on in one corner of the room and another, by talking, piano-strumming, and what not, I could have knocked their heads off!" (Patient no. 10700). Yet the responses of women to the asylum environment varied. Mrs. A, after campaigning for months to get released, wrote back to tell her doctor that she missed "all the noise and company" of the asylum (Patient no. 6712). But regardless of their response to the noisy asylum environment, one can assume that the level of constant noise would have been a new and different experience for most women who entered Essondale and New Westminster.

Another fact of patient life within the asylum was unpaid labour. Patient labour helped to offset costs and bring revenues into the asylum. In the early years of the period, revenues from patient work were significant; in 1910 a quarter of the entire patient maintenance budget was recouped. However, by 1935 costs had risen to $925,000 and revenues were less than $150,000 (Annual Reports 1934, X42–43; 1935, X56–57).

The fiscal benefits of patient labour found a convenient echo in the common medical belief that work itself constituted the best kind of therapy for the majority of patients. In fact, it appears that work was the only form of treatment that the majority of patients received at New Westminster and Essondale. In his 1912 annual report, Dr C.E. Doherty, the then asylum superintendent, wrote that both amusement and work were keys to the successful treatment of patients, adding that patients were encouraged to work in asylum shops and gardens and on the farm (Annual Report 1912, G8). Significantly, this use of work as the primary form of treatment employed at the asylum meant that the ability to be a cooperative, industrious worker was equated with good mental health.

Throughout the period under study, descriptions of patient work contained in the annual reports indicate clear differences between male and female labour.[8] While more attention was generally given to work done by men in the annual reports, particularly the activities of the Colony Farm at Essondale, the 1923 report provides a good description of the variety of work done by female patients:

The lady patients have also been occupied in productive occupations. Some have worked in the vegetable gardens and small fruits. The finishing room in the laundry occupies twenty. The tailor shop provides occupation for a score more, while the occupational room finds from eighty to ninety-five busily engaged everyday. Here much useful work is done ... Nearly 10,000 sheets were made, 100 table cloths, over 1,500 articles of clothing for free patients ... (Annual Report 1923–1924, P12).

We find that women often began their work career within the institution by performing domestic work on their own wards. Once a patient had proved to be a reliable and trusted worker, like Mrs. R who was moved to the tailor shop, she was moved off the ward (Patient no. 2670). At this point, female patients still performed what was essentially domestic labour, but in this instance they gained more physical freedom, a chance to do different kinds of work, and new opportunities to meet patients from other wards.

Gender-differentiated patient work served to reinforce the physical boundaries of the male and female communities at the two institutions. Men, if they proved to be cooperative patients and were not likely to try to escape, might be offered the opportunity of working at masculine occupations outside the asylum buildings – on the grounds or at Colony Farm, the institution's agricultural unit. The work set for female patients, however, restricted their movements to inside the institution or the immediate vicinity of the kitchen gardens.

Thus we find that the character of institutional life at New Westminster and Essondale shaped the lives of female patients in a number of ways. Gender-differentiated labour and living spaces meant
that there were essentially two separate communities within the asylum – one male and the other female. Institutional routine, too,
imposed a certain order on patient life; from the moment they
entered the asylum, female patients were expected to conform to
institutional criteria which were often impersonal. The institutional
setting, therefore, defined the spaces in which female patients moved
and the daily rhythm of their lives inside the asylum.

FEMINISING THE INSTITUTIONAL COMMUNITY: WOMEN'S CULTURE INSIDE THE ASYLUM

An initial sense of disorientation may have been resolved when a
patient began to establish a place for herself within the asylum community. We find that female patients brought into the institution
elements of the female culture in which they had worked and lived
outside the asylum and that they employed aspects of this culture
to cope with, and make personal, the impersonal world of the asylum.
The work patterns of female patients, forms of patient privilege and
resistence, the ways in which women interacted with their male doctors, and friendship between women, all indicate ways in which female patients were able to recreate the outside world inside the
asylum.

The gender differentiation of the institutional structure created
places and ways in which women's culture could assert itself. Patient
labour have helped to personalize the asylum for women. Female
patient labour did not simply represent exploitation, for the short
respite from the confinement of the ward which work offered might
well have had its own therapeutic value (Shortt 1986, 132). Moreover,
it has been argued that women have historically used familiar domestic rituals to comfort themselves in a strange, unknown environment (Conrad 1984, 9). Women at New Westminster and Essondale
found solace in performing household tasks. The kinds of work
which women performed as seamstresses, canners, and laundresses,
while limiting their sphere of activity, would also have allowed more
frequent and extended opportunities for patient interaction than
the work performed by men. Female friendships like the one between Mrs. T and Mrs. Y who were (the former's chart tells us)
"constant companions" likely grew over hours spent hemming sheets
and mending clothes (Patient no. 11228).

Women could also impose a kind of individuality on the asylum
environment by becoming either "good" or "bad" patients. S.E.D.

Shortt, looking at the London Asylum during an earlier period, writes of an asylum subculture, born out of the close daily contact between attendants and patients, "a relationship doubtless woven of rules broken, punishments dispensed, food denied or allocated, or liberties permitted" (Shortt 1986, 49). In addition to admittance procedures, there were codes of behaviour particular to the institutional community with which the new patient had to become familiar. New patients would have learnt the importance of complying with the daily routine of the institutions, the correct manner of addressing staff, and how to gain the special privileges that would give them more individual freedom. The case histories suggest that personal space and the freedom to move and make one's own choices were used by asylum staff and physicians to elicit good behaviour from patients.

Ward routine, the case records tell us, was a daily ritual of rising, dressing, eating, and working, broken on Sunday by church services and visitors. Women who cooperated with the routine were rewarded with extra privileges, which included working off the ward or the freedom to walk in the grounds alone in the evening or with a party in the afternoon. By 1920 part of the procedure for punishing and rewarding patients had become formalized into what was known as the parole system. Female patients throughout the period had been released on a probationary system whereby they were discharged into the care of a relative or friend; the patient case files tell us that, unlike many men (who were released on their own recognizance) women had to be signed out by a relative or friend. Under this new set of regulations, trusted patients were allowed out of the asylum for limited periods of time – an afternoon or a weekend. The common denominator of such privileges was a symbolic or real granting of freedom, privacy, and individuality. At New Westminster and Essondale, the end result of privileged patient status was most often discharge.

Often privileges given to a cooperative patient or punishments doled out to patients considered "difficult" had an importance which was only meaningful in the context of the asylum subculture. For example, Mrs. A's chart notes that "she was demanding certain privileges such as leaving cups in her room against the nurse's instruction which accounted for this trouble" (Patient no. 6712). Clearly, in this case, the cups left where they should not be were less important than disobeying a nurse's instructions; such small rules likely served to underscore lines of authority and power within the asylum. Mrs. N was considered a difficult case throughout her stay in the asylum because, as her physician noted at one point, "[she] is not conforming any better to Ward routine, discipline and self control" (Patient

no. 6196). Yet what was more significant was that the institutional
focus on discipline inevitably meant that the ability to conform to
asylum regulation was equated with good mental health.

The rewards system in place at New Westminster and Essondale
appears to have differentiated between men and women by making
it easier for men to leave the asylum. Similarly, we find that forms
of patient protest tended to reflect cultural patterns which were
gender specific. Escape and suicide were both characteristically male
forms of resistance, suggesting that the more cloistered life led by
female patients offered fewer opportunities for such actions. It is
also possible that this gender difference in the number of escapees
also related to differing male and female attitudes towards the atmosphere of the asylum. The interior, domesticated surroundings
of the institution, coupled with the fact that all patient labour was
unwaged, would not have seemed unfamiliar to most female patients.
For the men, it may have often seemed intolerable.[9]

One kind of protest most frequently employed by female patients
was the refusal of food.[10] A 1927 menu indicates that food at the
asylum was adequate but mundane and repetitive (BC Mental Health
Services Administration Records, Box 14, File 6). Patients who refused to eat would first be spoon-fed and then, if that failed, tube-
fed. One illustration of this process is Mrs. F, who believed that her
food at the asylum was poisoned. In 1923 and again the following
year she refused to eat and was tube-fed (Patient no. 6444). Elaine
Showalter's work on women and madness suggests that, because
women have a traditional link with food, women like Mrs. F may
have sought to express their anger through action centered around
the preparation and consumption of food (Showlater 1987, 162).

However, instances of female resistance in which women chose to
employ aspects of female culture to defy the institutional structures
were far from universal among the asylum populace. Rather, the
case histories which provide information about the relationship between female patients and their doctors suggest that an equal number of women attempted instead to recreate the gender dynamics
of the nuclear family, placing their doctor in the position of dominant, all-important male. Certainly, female patients were aware of
the role played by gender in the relationship which they had with
their doctor. The case histories chosen for this article suggest that
they expressed this awareness in a number of ways.

For some women, it appears that their attitude toward asylum
doctors was highlighted by a sense that these men could also be part
of the ideal of heterosexual romance. Miss J, for example, believed
that personal validation would come through marriage. The fact
that she turned to the main male presence in her world to fulfill the

role of a husband is not surprising. For example, in one of the copious letters which she wrote to her doctor, Miss J said, "Housework. It will become lovable when I have my own man and my own home ... And of all the classes of men I like none better than doctors" (Patient no. 10700).

This kind of patient-physician transference is scarcely surprising, for the psychiatrist is commonly characterized as an almost mystical figure of male authority and knowledge in female accounts of psychiatric treatment.[11] In Emily Holmes Coleman's fictionalized account of her stay in an American asylum during the 1920s, "Fathers, Husbands, Doctors, Gods emerge as enormous figures in her [Coleman's] mad world" (Callil and Siepman 1981, 3). Certainly, many female patients acknowledged the fact that the power held by the asylum doctors was similar to that held by other figures of male authority in their lives. Mrs. B, for example, several times referred to the asylum doctor as her "husband," while Mrs. F believed that her husband and doctor were conspiring against her (Patients nos. 6384 and 6444). Thus, for female patients, their relationship with their doctor was defined by both gender and power differences.

Similarly, relationships between female patients reflect the structure of the families which many women left behind when they entered the asylum. New friendships with other patients probably helped women feel at home in the asylum. Mrs. C, for example, wrote to tell her husband that she had a new friend, "There is a little girl here I love very dearly she is the image of my sister V" (Patient no. 10746). Perhaps, by finding a stand-in for a beloved sister, Mrs. C sought to recreate within the asylum a sense of kin and family, an important facet of female culture (Conrad 1983, 12–13).

The importance of female friendship is underscored by evidence that such friendships could last beyond the confines of the asylum. In 1931, more than a year after she left the asylum, Mrs. L wrote to a female friend who remained in the institution to say, "when you get well enough to go home I want you to come and see us. I have been thinking about you all so much and the happy times we had together. You sure are good company" (Patient no. 11228).

Incidents of female bonding, such as letters written to a friend left behind, are more frequent in the case histories of women and suggest that the social and emotional aspects of asylum life were of greater importance to women than men. Contemporary sociological material on heterosociability notes the affective nature of female friendships and the importance placed by women on their same-sex friendships (Woolsey 1987, 129–30). Similar bonding took place between women in New Westminster and Essondale.

Thus female culture manifested itself in a number of forms within the institutional community. In a variety of ways, women appear to have fostered cultural forms which helped them make the asylum a place that approximated the world of kin and work that they had left behind. Yet we cannot see this process as entirely positive, for the same adherence to family structure appears to have encouraged some women to replace familial figures of male authority with those of their physicians.

CONCLUSION

The institution was, in part, a replica of the larger society that surrounded it. A discussion of the female subculture and the experience of women as mental health patients in early twentieth-century British Columbia suggests that, when home and family were no longer variables, both the state and female patients themselves recreated outside society within the world of the asylum. For the patients, some things were simply givens – power and order imposed from above in the physical spaces set out for various kinds of patients and in the daily routine enforced through institutional discipline.

Yet within this ordered sphere, women patients affirmed their individuality and personal power through the creation of female-centered facets of the patient subculture. The case histories of female patients at the two institutions show that the institutionalized women made personal their surroundings, and they underline for us the importance of looking at how the weak create their own systems of order and power (Janeway 1981). We find that women imposed a more personalized character on the asylum community through the friendships they made, the work they performed and the ways in which they resisted institutional codes of behaviour.

NOTES

1 This work would not have been possible without the assistance and support of many individuals. To name a very few, I would like to express my appreciation to the staff at the Provincial Archives of British Columbia, the administration of the Riverview Mental Health Centre in British Columbia, Dr. Wendy Mitchinson, Greg Chwelos, Kileen Farrell, Lykke de la Cour, Michele Billung-Meyer and, especially Colin Coates.
2 It is beyond both the scope of this paper and the archival material available to ascertain whether subcultures based on class, ethnicity, or age existed within the female asylum community, although it is reason-

able to think that such differences did exist. Moreover, we can suppose that more institutional-centred criteria (an individual's state of health, the kind of labour performed, privileges received) may also have served to unite or divide patients.

3 The case histories which I have looked at show that women entered the asylum for a number of reasons: emotional distress might be a reaction to economic circumstances, childbirth, or domestic isolation. It is difficult and perhaps less than useful to look backward and pass judgement on the "sanity" of these women; my choice, therefore, has been to accept, whenever possible, the concerns and motivations of the women I study as genuine.

4 These figures are based on statistics culled from the Annual Reports of the medical superintendent in the *British Columbia Sessional Papers*. They represent the number of patients in residence at the close of the year. The cumulative total of patients treated for 1910 was 843, and for the 1934/35 fiscal year 3,721.

5 This paper does not deal with the committal patterns of women and men. For a discussion of gender and committals at New Westminster and Essondale see my MA thesis, Department of History, University of Waterloo.

6 A similar point is made by Daniel Francis (1981, 7).

7 All patient case files are from the Riverview Collection, G87024, PABC. For reasons of privacy, the patients' names are not used.

8 Shortt (1986, 132) also looking at the annual reports of the medical superintendent, makes this same point about the earlier period at London Asylum in Ontario. However, a closer analysis of patient case files indicates that male patients often began their asylum work careers by doing domestic work on their ward, suggesting that "male" labour was reserved for "good" male patients.

9 Elissa Gelfand (1983, 7), in her work on women's writings from French prisons, makes a similar suggestion, arguing that female prisoners are more likely to conform to the expectation that prisoners be passive. Men, however, tend to refuse this identification and are therefore more rebellious.

10 Interestingly, hunger strikes were also used by suffragettes imprisoned in England before World War I. Elaine Showalter (1987, 162) argues that these hunger strikes were, in fact, explicit statements of female anger and rebellion.

11 Judi Chamberlin's (1975) and Barbara Findlay's (1975) personal accounts of their experiences as psychiatric patients demonstrate that male therapists often have considerable power within the lives of their female patients, at times assuming the roles of father, husband or lover.

REFERENCES

Callil, Carmen and May Siepman 1981. "Introduction." In Emily Homes Coleman, *Shutter of Snow*. London: Virago.

Chamberlin, Judy 1975. "Struggling to Be Born." In Dorothy Smith and Sara J. David, eds., *Women Look at Psychiatry*. Vancouver: Press Gang Publishers.

Conrad, Margaret 1984. "Sundays Always Make Me Think of Home: Time and Place in Canadian Women's History." In Barbara Latham and Roberta Pazdro, eds. *Not Just Pin Money*. Victoria, BC: Camosun College Press.

Daly, Mary 1978. *Gyn/Ecology: The Metaethics of Radical Feminism*. Boston: Beacon Press.

Findlay, Barbara 1975. "Shrink! Shrank! Shriek!" In Dorothy Smith and Sara J. David, eds., *Women Look at Psychiatry*. Vancouver: Press Gang Publishers.

Francis, Daniel 1981. "The Development of the Lunatic Asylum in the Maritime Provinces." In S.E.D. Shortt, ed., *Medicine in Canadian Society: Historical Perspectives*. Montreal: McGill-Queen's University Press.

Gelfand, Elissa 1983. *Imagination in Confinement: Women's Writings from French Prisons*. Ithaca, NY: Cornell University Press.

Graham, Hilary and Ann Oakley 1981. "Competing Ideologies of Reproduction: Medical and Maternal Perspectives on Pregnancy." In Helen Roberts, ed., *Women, Health and Reproduction*. London: Routledge and Kegan Paul.

Grob, Gerald 1983. *Mental Illness and American Society, 1865–1940*. Princeton: Princeton University Press.

Janeway, Elizabeth 1981. *Powers of the Weak*. New York: Morrow Quill Paperbacks.

Lasch, Christopher 1973. *The World of Nations: Reflections on American History, Politics and Culture*. New York: Knopf.

Lebsock, Suzanne 1984. *The Free Women of Petersburg: Status and Culture in a Southern Town, 1784–1860*. New York: Norton.

McLaren, Angus 1986. "The Creation of a Haven for 'Human Thoroughbreds': Sterilisation of the Feeble-minded and the Mentally Ill in British Columbia." *Canadian Historical Review* 67(2): 127–49.

Mitchinson, Wendy 1987. "Gender and Insanity as Characteristics of the Insane." *Canadian Bulletin of Medical History* 4(2): 99–117.

Mitchinson, Wendy 1982. "Gynecological Operations on Insane Women: London, Ontario, 1895–1901." *Journal of Social History* 15(4): 467–84.

Shortt, S.E.D. 1986. *Victorian Lunacy: Richard M. Bucke and the Practice of Late Nineteenth-Century Psychiatry*. Cambridge: Cambridge University Press.

Showalter, Elaine 1987. *The Female Malady*. Harmondsworth: Penguin.

Woolsey, Lorraine K. 1987. "Bonds between Women and between Men. Part II: A Review." *Atlantis* 13(1).

Women, Work, and Well-Being
Les femmes, le travail, et le mieux-être

NANCY GUBERMAN

The Family, Women, and Caregiving: Who Cares for the Caregivers?

As governments shift the burden for much of the work of caring for dependent adults from public health and social services to unpaid labour in the home and community, women are being called upon to take up the slack. This paper addresses three questions raised by this new context: Why do women provide care? At what cost to themselves do women provide care? What are the alternatives to women's caregiving? Research supports the need for a multidimensional understanding of women's relation to caregiving, including psychological, social, and political factors. Whatever the motivating factors, women pay a high price for this caregiving in terms of the physical and emotional labour involved, the impact on their health, and the effects on their family and social life. While there is no easy answer to the questions of alternatives, one possible avenue is to separate the functions of caring for and caring about, with the former more widely carried out by the public sector.

La famille, les femmes et les soins:
qui prend soin des personnes qui prodiguent des soins?

Dans un contexte où les gouvernements sont en train de transférer une partie importante du travail de prise en charge des adultes qui dépendent des services sociaux et de santé publique vers la maison et la communauté, les femmes sont particulièrement interpellées. Cet article touche trois questions soulevées par cette situation: Pourquoi les femmes continuent-elles à assumer la prise en charge? À quel prix doivent-elles assumer cette prise en charge? Quelles alternatives pourraient être développées? Des recherches confirment la nécessité d'une compréhension multidimensionnelle du rapport des femmes à la prise en charge, compréhension qui tienne compte, à la fois, des facteurs psychologiques, sociaux et politiques. Peu importe les motivations qui les habitent, les

femmes payent un prix élevé en assumant ce travail. Cette situation implique un fardeau important et a des répercussions majeures sur leur
santé, ainsi que sur leur vie sociale et familiale. Finalement, s'il n'y a pas
de réponse facile à la question des alternatives, l'une des solutions possibles serait de séparer la dimension affective de la prise de charge et le
travail de soins quotidiens, lequel devrait être plus largement assumé par
les services publics.

Over the last fifteen years, there has been a renewed interest in the
family. No longer is the family seen as a pathological, problem-
generating system (as in many of the theories on the cause of mental
illness, juvenile delinquency, and so on) but rather as an ideal location
for caring and therapeutic activities. In contrast to the cold pecuniary
relations of the market, the family is seen as the setting for warmth
and unconditional love. It is the "haven in a heartless world."

Feminists have questioned the myth of the idealized family and
have shown that the emotions and well-being attributed to the family
exist – to the extent that they exist – mainly because of women's role
and place in that institution. As well, many would question whether
women's well-being is indeed being assured in the family, as attested
to by research on such subjects as violence against women in the
family, on the comparative well-being of married and single women,
on the concrete amount of work assumed by women in the family
and so on. Of particular interest to this paper is the increasing body
of research which reveals what most women have known for a long
time: that beyond assuming by far the major portion of caregiving
in our society, women also assume the responsibility of caring for
the dependent members of our society, be they children, the physically or mentally handicapped, the frail elderly, or the mentally ill.
To this research we can now add a number of studies that address
the question of the welfare of women who care for dependent adults
and that document the stresses and burdens of this work. Despite
the feminist indictment of the family, women are still investing heavily in this institution.

It is true that the family is almost the only legitimate place for the
expression of emotional needs, and that it offers the security of the
familiar and the rights and obligations that go along with a kin
relation. But the new myth of the family goes beyond that. The
simple fact of a biological tie supposedly enables families to answer
the universal needs of persons of both sexes, of all ages, and in all
situations. The counterpart of this myth is that institutional care is
to be avoided at all costs since institutions cannot provide the love
and caring which the family is thought to offer. Thus, shored up by

sociological criticism of asylums and the very real horror stories of patients in institutions paying the price for government cutbacks and inefficiency, families have increasingly decided, and even demanded, to care for dependent members themselves.

However, at the same time that families are expressing their desire to keep dependent adults out of institutions, the political and economic crisis of the welfare state has also led to renewed interest in the "community" and the family as the optimum loci for caring. This has resulted in shifts from paid caregiving by women in public health and social services to unpaid caregiving in the home and the community, putting both ideological and material pressures on families. Governments are calling on families to assume responsibility for themselves while these same governments bow out of many of the social commitments that they assumed in the 1960s and 1970s. In fact, one of the premises of recent government policies (particularly deinstitutionalization and home maintenance policies) is that families are capable of, willing to, and morally obligated to assume the care of their ill, elderly, and dependent members.

This complex situation creates a dilemma for women who on one hand, as mothers, daughters, sisters, and wives, are being told (and often genuinely feel) that they really ought to be providing care, and who on the other hand, as individuals, are touched by the feminist movement's demands for women's economic independence and choice of lifestyles.

Many intricate issues are at play here. In this presentation I would briefly like to address three of them: Why do women provide care? At what cost to themselves do women provide care? And what, if any, are the alternatives to women's caregiving?

WOMEN AND CAREGIVING

Interesting reflections on the question of women's relation to caregiving are to be found in work by both Hilary Graham and Clare Ungerson. Graham (1983) proposes that we understand caregiving as "both the identity and the activity of women in Western society." She thus calls for an analysis of women's relation to caregiving which collapses the dichotomy between the psychological and structural paradigms. The first of these paradigms sees caregiving as women's life work; it maintains that the qualities and characteristics required to care for someone are central characteristics of the female identity and are what distinguishes them from men. To be a woman is to care for others. The second perspective examines the social organization of caregiving in the context of the sexual division of labour. From this perspective, "caring emerges not so much as an expression of women's natural feelings of compassion and connectedness ... but as an expression of women's position within a particular kind of society in which the twin forces of capitalism and patriarchy are at work" (Graham 1983, 25). Echoing Graham, I feel that to understand fully women's work of caregiving, we must look at both the social and the psychological forces at play. To this, Ungerson (1983) adds that we must not neglect an analysis of state ideology and practice and their impact on family decisions with regard to caring for dependent members.

Recent research that I have been conducting on the conditions of caregiving for ex-psychiatric patients and frail elderly persons who have been deinstitutionalized (either sent out of institutions or kept out of them) tends to support the need for a multi-dimensional understanding of women's relation to caregiving.[1] While the research was not designed specifically to study the factors and motivations which led families first to assume the care of their dependent adults and then to assign this work to the adult women in the family, the data collected through open-ended semi-structured interviews does give us some understanding of why women provide care.

In all the families studied (seven caring for elderly parents, four caring for adult children who have spent time in psychiatric hospitals, and one caring for a husband diagnosed as schizophrenic), women were indeed assuming the major burden of caregiving. In most cases, situational factors were cited as the major reason for this division of labour. In three of the families, the daughters were looking after their ailing parents because they themselves were separated, divorced, or widowed and it seemed more natural that they, rather than their married sisters who had husbands to look after, be the ones to take care of their parents. As for their brothers, few of them were involved at all in the caregiving work. And as one woman explained to me, "When you're old, you go to your daughter's. It's rare that you go to your daughter-in-law's." Of course, if you have no daughters, then daughters-in-law do tend to assume this work, as was the case in one of the families. In the case of an ill or disabled husband, there is almost universal expectation that no matter what her situation, a wife will assume the full-time care of her husband should he become ill or disabled, and this was the case for the couple in our study. In two other cases, women were caring for their mothers despite marital and family obligations (adolescent children in the home) because they were only children.

This portrait confirms research that shows that marital status is an important predictor of involvement in caregiving (Brody and Shoonover 1986) – that is, single or divorced women are more likely to be involved than their married sisters. Other research demonstrates that sons involved in caregiving "do so by default in that there [is] no female alternative" (Horowitz 1985, 614). When sons are involved, the work of caring is shared by daughters-in-law. This is not the case with sons-in-law (Horowitz 1985).

Of course, the availability of non-married women in the family is more than just a situational factor. Comments throughout the interviews revealed that the women were aware of many of the psychological and social forces at play. Many other motives were stated or hinted at to explain why these women were providing care.

For example, a woman caring for her mother-in-law who was suffering from Alzheimer disease actually wanted to place her in an institution. One of the reasons she hesitated to do so was because she was afraid that her husband would accuse her of abandoning his mother and that this could conceivably lead to a divorce. A similar situation was present in two families caring for schizophrenic adult children. The mothers expressed some desire to institutionalize their children but hinted at their fears of the consequences of going against their husbands' wishes to keep the child at home. When asked why she did not place her mother in an institution, another woman replied:

She'd die right away. In any case, I can't place her. She's too healthy, they wouldn't accept her. They have a waiting list a mile long. Don't think I don't know how it works. I went through it with my father. She's not sociable, she wouldn't want to follow a schedule. She wasn't raised to accept an old folks' home. It's a different mentality from today's. People raised today are like that, but those of my mother's age never knew old folks' homes. She's always lived at home.

Other women told us:

When my mother became ill, I wanted to give her everything I could. But you can't give what you don't have. I don't have any money ... The only thing I could give her was to take her into my home ... Here, I spoil her like a child. She could never get such care elsewhere. When she's going to be institutionalized, she won't get such care.

She never got rid of us. I won't place her just to get rid of her. Residences are like prisons. They live by the bell. At such and such an hour you eat – hungry or not. If you're not hungry, too bad, you can't eat again until the next meal. There's no individual attention. Nobody comes to visit.

They're our parents. They gave us their youth. So why should I place her in a prison?

Well, he gets up early ... he works. If he'd look after his mother and get up nights with her and then get sick, How would we eat? The man has to work.

If I had the health for it, I would keep her. I would be happy to – because I love my husband, he's a good man.

I have no choice. I have to do it. They say it's my job. I'm caught, I'm trapped in this problem.

As we can see, a variety of factors are at play here, including internalized sex-role and filial obligation ideology, external pressures from other family members (real fears of losing their husbands if they refused to provide care), material conditions related to the sexual division of labour in the public and private spheres (husband's versus wife's earning power), lack of options (the only choice seems to be between the family or institutional care), and state practice (differential access to public services if there is a female relative "available" for caregiving, the bureaucratic impersonal care offered by public institutions, and so on).

But while these multiple factors have led these women to accept the care of dependent adults, they almost unanimously stated that they will never let their children assume such a burden when they themselves grow frail. Recently one even advised both a niece and a female cousin not to follow her example and assume care for their ailing mothers. "You'll regret it. You'll see, it's incredibly confining. Its a terrible responsibility," she told them.

THE COST OF CAREGIVING

As we have already stated, family care is a euphemism for women's caregiving, and this division of labour in the family has serious repercussions.

It is the mothers (biological, in the case of mentally ill children, and symbolic, in the case of daughters caring for frail elderly or handicapped husbands) who initiate, coordinate, and assume the tasks of physical care, providing housework and emotional support and making the necessary links with the formal service network.

It is the mothers who change the dirty diapers and wet sheets of incontinent parents, who do two or three loads of laundry a day, who get up three or four times a night to change a diaper or temper a crisis. It is the mothers who support a distraught schizophrenic child, fight to get doctors' appointments, yell at social workers for needed services.

In times of crisis, it is the mothers who control behaviour, administer medication, calm overexcited fathers, and generally take charge of tension management and intergenerational conflicts.

It is the mothers who worry that their dependent mothers, sons, or daughters have forgotten to turn off the stove, have fallen out of bed, or have had an outburst – this all the time, even when they are at work or when there is an alternative caregiver in the home.

It keeps me from sleeping. I'm afraid she'll wake up in the night and fall ... even at the hospital I called all the time so she wouldn't worry after I'd left for the day.

I don't want to go out because I'm always afraid she'll need me. I'm too worried when she's with a stranger.

At work, it is the mothers who fret over their sons' mental health or their retired husbands' frame of mind. "It hindered me in my work. I couldn't concentrate. I was worried about my husband's health."

Not only do women assume all the work of caring, but they are also profoundly marked by their feelings and by the reality of total responsiblity. This feeling (based on reality) of being the only one who can and ought to be there is expressed by statements of guilt or by rationalizations for the lack of participation on the part of other members of the family.

It is the mother who feels guilty about having caused her children's illness or about even thinking of placing her own mother in an institution.

You wonder, "What did I do?" For three or four years I would relive everything, often. His whole life, starting with my pregnancy through the birth, his early childhood, adolescence. I tried to figure out what had caused it. Maybe he was lacking something, maybe there was something I hadn't given him. Maybe I wasn't sensitive enough to see it coming. I'm very nervous.

I know that if I place her and she dies, I'll feel so guilty. It's funny. I'd rather she die here. I feel guilty.

And it is the mothers who excuse the others who don't care.

He works. Yesterday he got home for supper at 7:15. When he sits down at 7:15, he's tired. He works hard ... what can you expect. He won't lose his job to look after her.

We're six – three boys and three girls. There's one who lives in Florida. Okay, he can't come to see her every week. After that, I have another brother who lives nearby, but things were never easy for him at home so he's always cast mama aside. There's another one who lives with my sister. He'll come if mama needs anything, but other than that we don't see much of him ... I have two sisters. My mother stayed with one of them for awhile, but she exploited her, stole her things, and left her alone all the time. So my other sister begged me to take her.

But it is neither the physical and emotional labour nor the guilt which is the hardest burden to bear. The most severe effect of caring for a dependent adult appears to be that it is totally monopolizing and without respite, twenty-four hours a day, seven days a week, 365 days a year. Everyone interviewed, without exception, spoke about the serious restrictions that caregiving has on her social and family life. There is gradual isolation of the whole family, but particularly of the main caregiver. The main caregiver no longer goes out, no longer invites people over, no longer accepts invitations, because she cannot leave the dependent person alone and is too nervous about that person's unpredictable behavior to receive people or to have confidence in substitute care. "I thought it wouldn't be much work. But you're confined – I didn't think, you know, that I'd become a prisoner. I can't go out at all. Not at all."

Caring for a dependent adult also results in a state of extreme mental and physical fatigue which leads to health problems, insomnia, fear of "cracking," and even depression. There is constant fear and anxiety about the unpredicatble behavior of the dependent person.

At night she wakes up. She's wet. She's lost. I have to change her. I get up three, four times a night. My husband and I can't sleep. She smokes and we're afraid. I'm afraid she'll start a fire. It's stressful. I'm tired. I can't take it anymore.

With P., I'm too worried that something will happen if I go out for very long. I'm afraid she'll need me. I never know when there'll be a crisis, when I'll have to call an ambulance or the police. We're afraid of her violence.

Often these fears mark the beginning of a process of deterioration of the caregiver's own physical and mental health. She has difficulty concentrating, can't sleep, and suffers anxiety attacks or high blood pressure.

It started to affect my work. I couldn't concentrate. I was always worried. I was always on the verge of tears. I was really unhappy.I was completely exhausted. I suffered from insommnia. It was too much even to go to self-help meetings. I came back exhausted. I had a breakdown. It's the same for my friends – they're going through the same thing.

It's no joke. I'm going to end up having to see a psychiatrist. I can't keep all this in. I have to get out. I go for walks, long walks.

Caring for a dependent adult in the home also affects the climate in the family. The couple's relationship suffers from a lack of intimacy and from neglect because of the centrality of the caregiving.

We're not comfortable. We no longer feel at home. I would like to invite my sons for supper, but it's a problem. They have small children and they bother her.

As man and woman, for my wife and me, that's dead. It's finished because we can't do that. She would hear. You have nowhere to go in your own home. You have no intimate relations.

We don't have big arguments but it's always about his mother. I would like my husband to caress me, things like that. But living with his mother we can't. We've become distant. It's as if we were two strangers living together.

Another cost of caregiving is its impact on women's financial autonomy. Studies (Brody 1985, Wright 1983, Rimmer 1983) have shown that many women give up salaried work or switch to part-time work, with all the long-range financial repercussions that this change has on future earnings and pensions, in order to provide care. In my own research, two women had indeed stopped outside work and one feared she would have to leave her part-time job if her mother-in-law's condition deteriorated. "I worked before I took her in. I washed ceilings and walls. I was a cleaning lady. I stopped working. But those were my outings. It meant a lot to me. I like cleaning houses."

Quite clearly, caring for a dependent adult has serious repercussions on the caregivers. I have not of course counterbalanced this portrait with examples of the joys and rewards that caregiving can bring. But I must say that the positive side of the picture did not come out clearly in any of the interviews I did, nor is there much literature on the subject. The costs are so heavy that in the end they

greatly outweigh the joys, especially with the frail elderly. For as the
days, weeks and months go by, not only do the caregivers witness a
deterioration in their own and in other family members' physical
and mental health, but the situation of the person being cared for
only gets worse.

ALTERNATIVES

The question of alternative forms of caregiving must be posed in a
context in which the family is seen as the only alternative to institutional care. One of the main arguments for family care over professional care has been that families offer both caring for and caring
about, that their caregiving is imbued with a love and affectivity that
cannot be bought. Jarrett (1985) questions the assumption that home
care necessarily provides emotional closeness and even asks whether
affection is necessary to caregiving. He explains that it is only recently
in Western society that kinship relations have been seen as a set of
personal relations rather than as formal relationships with a system
of rights and obligations. This leads him to conclude that, as kin, we
may have obligations to dependent adults but we don't have to like
them nor the work we are doing for them.

Pushing his logic further, if caring about and caring for someone
can be separated and if caring for can be seen as an obligation, then
there is no specific reason why this labour cannot be performed by
non-family members. Aronson (1987) supports the idea that caring
about and caring for can be seen as two separate functions and
suggests that they could be divided between the private and public
spheres.

Another point to consider is the preference of dependent adults
for certain forms of care. Several studies (Wister 1985; Livre blanc
à l'égard des personnes handicapées 1977; Béland 1985) have found
that most dependent adults prefer privacy and independence to
living with and depending on their families. In the case of the elderly,
researchers (Matthews 1986, Roberto and Scott 1984–85, Bankoff
1983) have noted that contacts with widowed and single friends or
with siblings are more important than contacts with children. Lang
and Brody's 1983 study of three generations of women found that
the eldest cohort of women preferred paying a professional to help
them rather than relying on family or friends, especially if family
caregiving meant that a daughter had to leave paid employment.

All these factors taken together suggest that family care is neither
the preferred nor necessarily the preferable form of care for dependent adults. Innovations such as cooperative housing for the

elderly with on-site health care, food, and other services should obviously be examined. Finch and Groves (1982) for example, suggest the possibility of sheltered housing or residential homes for the elderly, sponsored by trade unions or benevolent associations.

But taking care out of the family does not guarantee that the caregiving will not be done by women. On the contrary, women make up the majority of the salaried and volunteer workers involved in caregiving. Cooperative residential housing with in-house services using low-paid female labour does not really solve the problem. As well, as Finch (1983) points out, we must take into account powerful cultural rules which operate in the sphere of caregiving. Most women who are physically highly dependent prefer to be cared for by women, and the majority of the elderly are, of course, women.

As we can see, there are many Catch-22s involved in the issue of women and caregiving and it is not within the scope of this presentation to deal with these. It is important, however, at a time when the crisis of the welfare state affects both paid careers through cutbacks and voluntary and domestic caregivers through new interest in family and community care, to become aware of the scope of the problem. One can hope that new and creative strategies will come out of our collective exchanges, strategies which collectivize the problem while at the same time taking into account the well-being of both the caregivers and the cared for.

NOTES

1 A part of this research was done in collaboration with Pierre Maheu and Henri Dorvil and was financed by the Commission d'enquête sur les services de santé et les services socieux. This article was originally published in *Resources for Feminist Research/Documentation sur le recherche féministe* 17(3) (June 1988).

REFERENCES

Aronson, J. 1986. "Care of the Frail Elderly. Whose Crisis? Whose Responsibility?" *Canadian Social Work Review* 45–58.

Bankoff, E.A. 1983. "Social Support and Adaptation to Widowhood." *Journal of Marriage and the Family* 45: 827–39.

Brody, E.M. and C.B. Shoonover 1986. "Patterns of Parent-Care When Adult Daughters Work and when They Do Not." *The Gerontologist* 26(4): 372–81.

Brody, E.M. 1985. "Parent Care as a Normative Family Stress." *The Geron-tologist* 25(1): 19–29.

Finch, J. 1983. "Community Care: Developing Non-sexist Alternatives." *Critical Social Policy* 9: 6–18.

Finch, J. and D. Groves 1982. "By Women, for Women: Caring for the Frail Elderly." In *Women's Studies International Forum*, 5(5): 427–38.

Graham, H. 1983. "Caring: A Labour of Love." In J. Finch and D. Groves, eds., *A Labour of Love*. London: Routledge and Kegan Paul.

Gouvernement du Québec 1977. *Livre blanc, proposition de politique à l'égard des personnes handicapées.*

Horowitz, A. 1985. "Sons and Daughters as Caregivers to Older Parents: Differences in Role Performance and Consequences." *The Gerontologist* 25(6): 612–17.

Jarrett, W.H. 1985. "Caregiving within Kinship Systems: Is Affection Really Necessary?" *The Gerontologist* 25(1): 5–10.

Lang, A. and E.M. Brody 1983. "Characteristics of Middle-aged Daughters and Help to Their Elderly Mothers." *Journal of Marriage and Family* February: 193–201.

Matthews, A.M. 1986. "Widowhood as an Expectable Life Event." In J. Crawford, ed., *Aging in Canada: Social Perspectives*. Don Mills, Ontario: Fitzhenry and Whiteside.

Rimmer, L. 1983. "The Economics of Work and Caring." In J. Finch and D. Groves, eds., *A Labour of Love*. London: Routledge and Kegan Paul.

Roberto, K.A. and J.P. Scott 1984–85. "Friendship Patterns Among Older Women." *International Journal of Aging and Human Development* 19: 1–10.

Ungerson, C. 1983. "Why Do Women Care?" In J. Finch and D. Groves, eds., *A Labour of Love*. London: Routledge and Kegan Paul.

Wister, A.V. 1985. "Living Arrangement Choices among the Elderly." *Canadian Journal on Aging* 4: 127–44.

Wright, F. 1983. "Single Careers: Employment, Housework, and Caring." In J. Finch and D. Groves, eds., *A Labour of Love*. London: Routledge and Kegan Paul.

LESLIE BELLA

An Exploration of the Work Women Do to Produce and Reproduce Family Leisure

The concept of leisure is androcentric. Particularly problematic is the literature on "family leisure," which implies that all family members have leisure together. Women work to create leisure (for example Christmas) for their families. Interviews show the impact of childhood memories of the production of Christmas by mothers and grandmothers and the influence of these memories on women's expectations of themselves and their families. Women see the production of Christmas as reaffirming ties to the past and to friends and family in the present. Christmas was perceived as a process of reproducing – as reproductive labour. Also, Christmas told people they were affirmed or cared about. In short, women saw Christmas in terms of relationality. New patterns reduce the physical work for some women today, but the emotional work of creating the positive social environment needed for enjoyable family leisure remains significant.

Une exploration du travail des femmes pour
organiser et reproduire les loisirs familiaux

La notion de loisir est axée sur les hommes. Les textes qui portent sur les "loisirs familiaux" sont particulièrement problématiques puisqu'ils supposent que tous les membres de la famille passent ensemble des heures de loisir. Pourtant ce sont les femmes qui travaillent à la création des loisirs (à l'occasion de Noël par exemple). Des entrevues révèlent que les souvenirs d'enfance des préparatifs que faisaient leurs mères et leurs grands-mères pour Noël ont une influence sur les attentes des femmes par rapport à elles-mêmes et à leur famille. Les femmes considèrent la préparation de cette fête comme un moyen de renouer avec le passé et avec leur famille et leurs relations d'amitié du présent. Elles perçoivent Noël comme un processus ou un travail de reproduction. Noël dit également aux gens qu'on les aime et qu'ils sont importants. Bref, les femmes envisagent Noël sous l'aspect des rapports humains. De nouveaux procédés réduisent le travail physique de certaines femmes, mais le travail émotionnel pour créer le contexte social positif nécessaire pour que les loisirs familiaux soient agréables demeure important.

INTRODUCTION

A critique of the androcentric bias in leisure theory and research has highlighted the prevalence of sexist language in the leisure literature and the androcentric nature of the concept of leisure (Bella 1986; Bella 1990). Two particular problems with leisure research, familist assumptions and reliance on time-budget studies have been identified. Time-budget studies tend to focus on activities and ignore the relational context which gives meaning to those activities. These studies neglect the multilayered nature of women's lives, in which several activities are engaged in simultaneously. Also, familist assumptions underlie studies of "family leisure," which tend to ignore the reality that family leisure must be organized by someone. Family leisure is in all probability women's work. Research to reveal the work women do to create family leisure will allow us to understand the relational context of that experience.

The work women do to create family leisure and the meaning of that work are explored here. A family Christmas is generally expected to be a happy holiday. Even the chores associated with producing Christmas are presented as being part of the "fun." My own experience, however, suggests that the holiday required hard work and that happiness was not always attainable.

Christmas can be excruciatingly painful. Other women reported similarly ambivalent and emotion-laden reactions. Christmas seemed to epitomize and bring into focus both the invisible emotional work and visible physical work women do to create happy experiences in their families.[1] This preliminary and limited study of the production and reproduction of Christmas began with a number of informal discussions with women and in an attempt to record my own experience. This led to the development of a topical outline for interviews with a larger group of women. An interviewer (Candas Dorsey) conducted twelve in-depth interviews, using this guide as a starting point. The results were transcribed, and a simple form of content analysis was used to identify major themes. An initial draft was shared with groups of women and confirmed and enriched by their experience.

Christmas, we found, is not merely produced but consciously reproduced. Women describe golden memories of the Christmases

produced by their grandmothers, mothers, and other female relatives. These earlier experiences influence women's expectations of
themselves and their families in producing Christmas today. The
women also confirm the significance of this celebration in establishing and reaffirming loving family relationships. However, the workload is frustrating, and menfolk are usually uncomprehending and
unsupportive. Women experience tension and pain, and Christmas
sharpens divisions in families already experiencing unhappiness.
Some have moved beyond this pain, and arrived at new family patterns which share the responsibility. But other women remain trapped, as much by their own values as by those of a spouse or child.
They seem to have an internalized demand to reproduce a Christmas
as golden and as happy as the celebrations presided over by their
grandmothers.

THE CHRISTMAS OF OUR FOREMOTHERS

Most women have some early memories of magical Christmases. A
grandmother was often the centrepiece of these memories, performing roles and setting standards against which later Christmases
are compared. Grandmothers were "the centre of everything," "the
key," "doing 99.9 per cent of the work." They cooked, cutting min-
iature noodles by hand and perking coffee before anyone else was
up. They were "the embodiment of hospitality," making Christmas
"magically happen."

After a grandmother's death, Christmas never seemed quite the
same, not authentic. However, mothers generally accepted most of
the responsibility, becoming the centre of the universe at Christmas.
Even women employed outside the home would do everything: the
social organization to bring everyone together; the cleaning; the
decorating; and the "wonderful meal, which was a good, good part
of it." One woman described her mother's role in the production of
Christmas this way:

She was the one who saved and folded wrapping paper for next year. She
was the one who decorated the tree, because she is very artistic. She had
made these special felt brick things to cover the wall so that it would look
like we had a chimney when we didn't. She had done all the cooking and
all that kind of stuff. There were treats first thing in the morning, and you
know there was this great big breakfast.

Women, including aunts and other female relatives took the brunt
of the responsibility, and one woman usually had a pivotal role in
planning and implementing the celebration. Often this work seemed

invisible and Christmas would "magically appear" as it did in grandmother's time. Most women interviewed, however, are now aware
of the work that their mother and other women had done and of
its significance. Most of the specific tasks associated with Christmas
had been women's work.

The orchestration of gift exchanges, for example, was mother's
responsibility. Gift shopping was a "great to-do," involving carefully
planned expeditions with children to find presents for everyone to
give everyone else. Mothers also supervised children's efforts to
make homemade gifts and escorted children to visit Santa Claus.
Women were in charge of stocking stuffing and leaving out "a little
table full of treats for Santa and his reindeers." Gift wrapping was
also women's work, with presents looking "like they were a work of
art." And when presents were unwrapped, "who cleaned up the
mess? My Mom!"

Cooking would begin weeks, even months, ahead. Cookies would
be baked and frozen, with "shortbreads one weekend and her al-
mond crescents the next." Children would sample everything as it
was made, building up their anticipation of the big event. There
would be long days in the kitchen just before Christmas, "mixing
coleslaw and that sort of thing." One mother "had not slept all the
night before because she was busy baking."

One woman compared her mother's family Christmas to annual
report time at her father's office. Her mother had been responsible
for "any of the contact that was established annually" by the family,
including seasonal hospitality and Christmas cards. This concern for
people and relationships is reflected in the following excerpt:

I remember Mom sitting and writing hundreds – it seemed like thousands
– of Christmas cards, back in the days when Christmas cards were two cents
for postage ... and she sent Christmas cards to every single member of the
family, everyone she knew, everyone she had ever known, any of Dad's
business friends. There would be just piles and piles of cards ... and writing
forever.

In most instances a father's role was restricted and specific, with
overall coordination remaining women's work. A father might have
written addresses on Christmas card envelopes or "helped in the
kitchen, peeling potatoes." But "Mom was really organizing it." The
only things that some men did was serve the drinks and carve the
turkey. The rest of the time they would "just sit downstairs and get
waited on." Quite a few men accepted responsibility for picking up
the tree and (more often) for "the electrical stuff" like putting the
lights on. However, several interviewees remembered their fathers

as having a sense of the Christmas spirit and being able to communicate it to others, even if they didn't actually do much physical work. One father had a special role bringing home the "great wonderful present that was sort of the present to beat all presents." Another was "the anchor in the middle of this storm and flurry," which really "worked out" for everybody. One father was clearly the source of the Christmas spirit, supplying "the dream quality that the children need. He was like the green elf, and he would package up these little things and wrap things for our stockings."

REPRODUCING OUR OWN FAMILY CHRISTMAS

These patterns, remembered from their grandparents in their early childhood or observed in their mothers and fathers, influence women's expectations of Christmas and of themselves in the present. Some women consciously try to reproduce the Christmases of their childhood. The concern for continuity and for retained ties to the past remains important. For the women interviewed, Christmas is not merely produced but reproduced. They try to do it the way it was when they were children, with everything just the same. The sense of continuity was crucial to a good Christmas, allowing one to trace one's roots to mothers and grandmothers and to remember one's own childhood, since many good memories have to do with Christmas.

The creation of attractive decorations, table settings, gift wrapping, and clothing are all an important part of this sense of continuity. Everything has to be "very special," with a table set beautifully with flowers and "grandfather's silverware." Some women try to recreate the "Christmas-card Christmas" that they believe their children expect and to produce it magically as a surprise. But inevitably they feel they have somehow fallen short of maintaining all the Christmas traditions, and they feel guilty.

For many women there is clearly a deep sense of obligation to reproduce Christmas as it had been in their childhood. The concept of reproductive labour used by Marxists in their analysis of the work women do in families to reproduce the work force (Dickinson and Russell 1986) seems particularly appropriate to the work done by these women in reproducing Christmas. Whether specific traditions are continued or abandoned in favour of a more relaxed celebration requiring less work, all the women interviewed spoke of the meaning and significance of the Christmas celebrations to themselves and their families. All the different components of Christmas were seen as symbolizing, reaffirming, or reinforcing the ties between family members and close friends. To these women, the family Christmas is about people and the quality of relationships between them, not about specific symbols.

It's the time when people stop and think about who they are, and it's an important time. People start to think about themselves, and gatherings, and letting their defences down.

Communication is important. It's a time of year when you can say, indirectly or directly, "I really care about you" and "you mean a lot to me" and "you've enhanced my life."

I learned that the joy of Christmas (or lack of it) is not in where you are but who you spend it with and the love that exists among those people. I have to have my family there, and the more time I can spend with them the better.

A "real" Christmas is one with good happy relationships, an occasion. That would be the key – being together with people that you really love, and having time to do that. Everybody is putting a little more effort into getting along with each other. They are on their best behaviour; they're trying to be humorous, friendly, and warm.

It ought to be one of the few times when people can actually get together and enjoy each other's company, that haven't been able to see each other for a long time because of life and work and so on. You look forward to the arrival of friends and relatives that you haven't had a chance just to be jovial with. It should have the feeling of a party, except better. Meaningful is the key word. It isn't the ritual per se, but a connection with somebody.

You sort of knock down the barriers a bit and people just relax and enjoy one another's company, as one human being to another. That's probably what makes Christmas special.

Togetherness, family being together, health which came to be a very valued commodity over time, if everyone was there and they were together and healthy; thoughtfulness, not so much expense or whatever, but more in-vention and attention to who people were at that time. Warmth, I guess. Strong connections with people, be they your natural birth family or adopted families or really strong friendships or whatever – those basic people things, that's what makes it [Christmas] for me.

What I really loved about Christmas at my grandmother's was that there was such a big body of people. You belonged to all these people – you could sit on the lap of all these people – they all gave you presents and you could give them little things, and they'd get excited about their little presents. So you felt as if you belonged. There was this incredible sense of belonging to a long history of people celebrating. All the way from Scotland, you know, and here we were.

The specific traditions of Christmas are valued because they symbolize this connectedness and relationship between people, including the connectedness with absent grandparents and parents. Food, for example, is more than nourishment, it is "something that you do together, that brings everybody enjoyment." The meal is an acknowledgement that says "you matter."

Gifts also have meaning in term of relationships to others. Even small or homemade gifts have really to fit the person. Women try to find gifts to "make someone feel that they are cared about," that their aspirations are recognized and advanced. Some women prowl the stores for hours and hours, for the present that was special and perfect for a particular person.

So women try to create a Christmas in which people feel affirmed and cared about and in which relationships are strengthened. Sometimes this involves peacekeeping, or ensuring that the atmosphere of cordiality and warmth persists. Women feel they have to push things under the carpet, to keep up a good front, to make sure people are fed and happy. Some women are on tenterhooks, particularly if Christmas celebrations tend to lead to excessive drinking.

While most women expect to carry the Christmas traditions of their birth family into their own marriage, a number described their frustration at their own and their spouse's inability to recreate the warmth that they had valued in the Christmas traditions of their own birth family. Christmastime in one marriage was "horrible," and another common-law relationship produced several "bad Christmases."

It was the first Christmas that I really didn't feel happy about. Mom and Dad came out to visit us, but there was just the four of us and it was very awkward and we didn't have a lot of money. We had to make paper strings for the trees – it just didn't feel right. We basically didn't have any friends in Victoria, so it was really just the four of us.

One husband tried to buy rather than bake Christmas foods, "to minimize the real work." To his wife, this cheapens the whole thing. Another man complained that society says "you have to buy a present," whereas his wife gets "really mad" with him because she loves

Christmas and he "just couldn't be bothered." She gets Christmas presents for the cat, but he "gets no fun out of it." He gives people things he has scrounged or has not used for a while. She could "kill him" for this, because "you don't give somebody something you're trying to get rid of." In-laws were also criticized for the lack of warmth in their traditions. They would "ho-hum" over their presents and exchange ritual kisses on the cheek, but without any feeling of celebration. Women complained of utilitarian Christmases, non-events, without that special spirit of Christmas.

Some Christmases have become less meaningful because the woman who had played the pivotal role decided not to do so any more. One woman just gave up when she went back to work. Another woman had a nervous breakdown "due very largely to the fact that every single Christmas celebration, Easter celebration, and so forth was left entirely to her." Now she refuses to lift a finger at Christmas, even to wipe a dish.

Even when she hasn't done anything, she gets infuriated – is very testy – because Christmas for her now brings back memories of utter resentment towards the rest of us, even the kids. And it's ruined it for her. She hates Christmas now, and she'll never lift a finger to help out again.

Other women also become angry and "choked up" over the work required of them (or that they required of themselves) at Christmas. One became so angry at working overtime to produce Christmas that she couldn't even eat the meal she had prepared. Another finds it very tiring, and comments she would be very happy "if we didn't have to celebrate the birth of Jesus." Another hates Christmas so much that she has a difficult time talking about it.

Sharing the work helps reduce this frustration. The women interviewed were more likely to be involved in sharing the workload than their mothers or grandmothers had been, partly because they were more likely to be employed outside the home. In one family with two employed parents, the division of labour is very unclear. Another woman works the night shift, so Christmas dinner is produced by her father and stepmother. In another household, the husband is secondary cook, preparing vegetables under supervision. Cooking is now more likely to be shared, with children accepting responsibility for washing and drying dishes, tidying the house, or cleaning the bathroom. In some households different family members contribute dishes for the meal. One woman contributes "the chocolate slice and lemon butter" because those are the things she likes to make. Another receives traditional pasta and braided bread

and other things so that she does not have to make them all. In one
family

Our dinner is really fun, because D's best at gravy; P usually sets the table,
because he always makes sure that everything's just so on the table. Everybody's got a role because I don't want the fatigue that I discovered could
creep up if you would try and do too much.

However, in some families the division of responsibilities is still
very traditional:

My husband and I share. He doesn't know how to cook, so I cooked Christmas dinner. I didn't cook very many cookies, because I am trying to lose
weight. He went out and picked up any alcohol we needed. He picked out
the Christmas tree, brought home and decorated it. He made it quite nice
and put up ornaments.

Some men would participate more but are covertly dissuaded by
women who want perfection rather than participation: "If I ask him
to wrap the gifts, because that's part of the work and it takes time,
they aren't wrapped very nicely."
    Some women have clearly redesigned the roles in their families
so that the work of organizing the family Christmas (and one sus-
pects, family leisure generally) no longer rests totally on their shoul-
ders. However, most of those interviewed continue to work very
hard at the physical chores associated with producing Christmas.
Even those women who share the physical work with others continue
to assume responsibility for overall coordination and for creating
the positive emotional climate. Women continue to do the less visible
emotional and organizational work required to reproduce Christmas. Most women still tend to be responsible for the overall coordination even though "the tasks are divided up a little bit more." In
only one instance was the social convenor role shared with a male
family member. He was described as the social manager, producing
with gusto a breakfast of pancakes with strawberries and whipped
cream.

CONCLUSION

An exploratory study of the work women do to produce family
leisure has shown that when they were children women had experienced Christmas with joy and pleasure – as leisure. But for adult
women in families the organization of leisure for the family clearly

involves work as well as leisure. Some of it is pleasurable, but it is still sufficiently tiring that some women experience significant fatigue, anger, and frustration. No women to whom I spoke or who was interviewed was emotionally neutral. Many had strong negative feelings, even though they also spoke warmly of the rewards in seeing a loving family sharing a celebration together. While some had achieved a shared responsibility within the family, others continued to assume all responsibility. The concept of family leisure prevalent in the literature clearly needs to be reexamined to reveal which family members must work in order that others experience leisure. This exploratory study suggests that family leisure is women's work.

All the women interviewed work hard to reproduce Christmas. Some continue to work physically hard, reproducing the symbols associated with the ritual celebrations. The symbols, for these women, are significant in affirming and maintaining their bonds with family members, past and present. Even the specific symbols are understood in terms of the relationships they are intended to strengthen and the people they are intended to affirm. A time-budget study would reveal the specific activities in which these women engage in reproducing Christmas, but such studies would not reveal the meaning of those activities to the women involved or to their families. A time-budget study cannot show that a woman produces a Christmas dinner because she hopes it will tell her family members that she thinks they are important. Nor will such a study show the significance of the mealtime rituals in remembering a lost childhood or parents and grandparents that have died. The meaning of activity – its significance – is invisible to such methods.

I have suggested elsewhere (Bella 1986; Bella 1990) that the concept of leisure itself is inappropriate for understanding what happens in families. This study of family Christmas illustrates this point. The meaning and significance of Christmas celebrations and associated activities can best be understood in terms of relationships between people (Wine 1982) and reproductive labour (Dickinson and Russell 1986) rather than in terms of a sterile dichotomy between work and leisure. Women in particular value Christmas because of the opportunity it provides to reinforce and reaffirm the loving relationships between family members. Women know that physical work is required, and many now work out ways of sharing that work. The organizational work (dividing up the chores, planning the menu) and the emotional work (peacekeeping, emotional support) required for a successful Christmas are less visible and therefore more difficult to share. I hope that this paper will provide an initial insight into that invisible work.

NOTES

1 Other specific celebrations might include Thanksgiving, birthday parties, weddings, anniversaries, summer holidays, or Sunday suppers reuniting grown children with their parents, or the organization of less elaborate family leisure such as trips to the swimming pool, playground, library, restaurant, or circus.

REFERENCES

Bella, Leslie 1986. "Androcentrism in Leisure Theory and Research," CRIAW, Winnipeg.
Bella, Leslie 1990. "Beyond Antrocentrism: Women and Leisure." In E.L. Jackson and T.L. Burton, eds., *Understanding Leisure and Recreation: Mapping the Past, Charting the Future*. Pennsylvania: Venture Publishing.
Dickinson, James and Bob Russell 1986. *Family, Economy and State: The Social Reproduction Process under Capitalism*. Toronto: Garamond.
Wine, Jeri Dawn 1982. "Gynocentric Values and Feminist Psychology." In Angela Miles and Geraldine Finn, eds., *Feminism in Canada: From Pressure to Politics*. Buffalo: Black Rose.

CAROLINE ANDREW, CÉCILE CODERRE, ET ANN DENIS

Le mieux-être et le travail: contradiction ou compatibilité

Cet article traite des rapports entre le travail et le mieux-être chez un groupe de femmes gestionnaires. Les auteures explorent l'idée qu'un des éléments importants de satisfaction tient à la compatibilité entre la vie au travail et les autres dimensions de la vie. Deux niveaux de compatibilité sont examinés dans l'article. D'abord, bien que le travail de ces femmes soit accaparant, il leur laisse tout de même la possibilité d'une certaine vie hors travail. Deuxièmement, cet emploi n'est pas incompatible avec leur identification comme femmes ou, plutôt, les femmes-cadres qui font l'objet de l'études ne se sentent pas obligées d'oublier qu'elles sont des femmes pour réussir dans leur carrière.

Well-Being and Work:
Contradictory or Compatible?

This article examines the relations between work and well-being for a group of women managers. The authors explore the idea that one of the important elements that leads to satisfaction is a high level of compatibility between life at work and other aspects of life. Two levels of compatibility are looked at in the article. First of all, although the work done by these women is demanding, the constraints of work permit the possibility of a certain life outside work. Secondly, the work of women managers is not incompatible with their identification as women or, perhaps more accurately, the women managers studied do not feel obliged to deny that they are women in order to be successful in their careers.

Dernièrement, une série d'articles parus dans les journaux – surtout de sources américaines – indiquaient que les femmes elles-mêmes critiquaient un certain type de carrière. Ces articles font référence à des études qui démontrent qu'un nombre important de femmes qui réussissent dans leurs carrières commencent à se poser des questions et, plus encore, commencent à quitter ces carrières « réussies » pour s'occuper de leurs enfants ou de leur famille. La plupart de ces études semblent insister sur le fait que ces femmes considèrent qu'il est impossible de combiner carrière et responsabilités familiales d'une façon satisfaisante et, dans l'impossibilité de faire plusieurs choses à la fois, décident de se définir par rapport à un seul rôle: celui de mère.

Ces articles véhiculent donc cette vision de l'échec d'une carrière réussie pour les femmes ou, peut-être plus précisément, la vision de l'échec d'une définition multidimensionnelle de la vie des femmes. Faire plusieurs choses à la fois, avoir diverses définitions de ses rôles sociaux, tout cela est impossible car la carrière semble prendre trop de place. Travail et mieux-être sont incompatibles, non pas en soi, mais parce que le fait d'accorder trop d'importance au travail implique qu'on ne peut pas donner suffisamment d'importance à ses responsabilités familiales ou à d'autres dimensions de la vie. Dans ces mêmes études, réussir une carrière de type professionnel implique que le travail devient trop accaparant. Ces femmes ne veulent pas renoncer au rôle familial et se voient donc obligées de renoncer à leur carrière, voire de l'abandonner.

Cette idée de l'incompatibilité ou de l'harmonie entre différents aspects de la vie des femmes nous a paru importante à explorer. Dans cette communication, nous voulons présenter certaines réflexions suscitées par une recherche menée auprès de 214 femmes gestionnaires des secteurs public et privé au Canada. Nous pouvons parler d'un groupe de femmes ayant des carrières de type professionnel qui sont, si nous les comparons avec le profil global des femmes sur le marché du travail, réussies. Ces femmes sont, en général, très satisfaites des leur situation. Dans leur cas, nous pouvons dire que travail et mieux-être sont plus que compatibles. Le travail est une des sources principales dans l'évaluation de leur mieux-être. Dans cette présentation, nous voulons reprendre cette question de la contradiction ou de l'incompatibilité entre les différentes dimensions de la vie et ce, dans le cas de travailleuses. Nous voulons aussi voir quelles formes de conciliation entre les exigences d'un travail de type professionnel et les autres dimensions de la vie elles ont inventoriées. Si elles sont en général très satisfaites de leur travail et si, par ailleurs, elles ont des postes d'un niveau important de responsabilités, il devient intéressant de voir comment elles ont concilié leur carrière avec les autres dimensions de leur vie. Leur mieux-être doit être en fonction de ces possibilités de conciliation.

L'objectif original de notre enquête n'était pas du tout de saisir le mieux-être de ces femmes gestionnaires mais plutôt d'analyser leur cheminement de carrière et particulièrement des interrelations entre les études, le travail et la vie familiale et personnelle. Le questionnaire qui préparait les entrevues est donc centré sur le milieu de travail et sur la vie au travail. D'autres dimensions de la vie sont explorées, mais surtout en relation avec le travail. De plus, le questionnaire ne touchait que très accessoirement la satisfaction au travail. Il traitait surtout des différents postes occupés, de la logique des changements de poste et des expériences comme avec des mentors ou des réseaux informels. Il portait donc plus sur les dimensions objectives du travail que sur les dimensions subjectives, telles la satisfaction. Mais dans cette communication nous allons tenter de relier certains aspects de la vie de nos répondantes qui, selon nous, peuvent expliquer leur satisfaction au travail. Avant d'aborder de plein pied cette question, il faut donner quelques précisions sur l'échantillon et établir ce que nous entendons par la « satisfaction ».

Nous avons interviewé 214 femmes qui occupaient des postes de gestionnaires intermédiaires et supérieures dans les secteurs privé et public au Québec et en Ontario. Pour le secteur privé, nous avons choisi de grandes sociétés qui ont leur siège social à Montréal ou à Toronto. Pour le secteur public, nous avons choisi les fonctions publiques du Québec, de l'Ontario et celle du gouvernement fédéral. Les interviews furent réalisées durant l'été et l'automne 1985. Très peu de gestionnaires ont refusé de participer à la recherche et nous sommes très reconnaissantes envers les répondantes de leur coopération.

Pour décrire l'opinion des femmes sur leur carrière, nous utilisons un nombre d'indices qui nous permettent de situer l'importance accordée à leur travail par les gestionnaires. Nous devons d'ailleurs signaler que la notion de carrière est une notion importante, mais qui a une signification parfois ambiguë. D'une part, nos prétests ont démontré que les femmes ne considéraient pas leur travail simplement comme un emploi, mais vraiment plus comme une carrière. Par contre, certaines de nos répondantes ont refusé de parler de « carrière », se disant opposées à devenir carriéristes. Tout au long du questionnaire, les femmes ont insisté sur le contenu du travail plutôt que sur le niveau hiérarchique de leur poste.

Pour illustrer l'importance accordée au travail, nous allons décrire les réponses données par les femmes sur leur futur cheminement de carrière, les facteurs auxquels les femmes accordent le plus et le moins d'importance, et la satisfaction au sujet de leur cheminement de carrière. Selon tous ces indices les femmes sont satisfaites de leur travail et en envisagent le développement.

Nous avons demandé aux femmes comment elles définissent leur futur cheminement de carrière, puis quel poste ou type de poste elles aimeraient occuper dans cinq ans (Tableau 1). La majorité des gestionnaires indiquent qu'elles veulent rester dans le même type de travail. Moins de 10% ont indiqué qu'elles envisageaient de changer radicalement de travail dans les cinq prochaines années et un nombre à peu près égal ont déclaré qu'elles n'avaient vraiment pas de plan défini. Toutefois ces pourcentages peuvent donner une impression exagérée du nombre de femmes qui recherchent un changement important dans leur milieu de travail. Puisque la moitié de celles qui envisagent un changement radical vont prendre leur retraite au cours de ces cinq ans, ce changement n'est donc pas nécessairement un choix. De plus, celles qui répondent qu'elles n'ont pas de plan clairement défini ne sont pas nécessairement mal à l'aise dans leur travail. Leur réponse correspond plutôt à une prise de position vis-à-vis de l'idée d'un cheminement planifié.

Ainsi 82% des répondantes envisagent de rester dans le même type de travail. Dans la plupart des cas, elles envisagent les cinq prochaines années avec optimisme, car la majorité ont répondu soit dans le sens d'un mouvement vertical (39%), soit dans le sens d'un développement de leur carrière défini en fonction du contenu du travail mais généralement, au moins implicitement, impliquant un progrès dans la carrière (22%). En fait la très grande majorité de nos répondantes n'envisageaient pas du tout de quitter le milieu de la gestion dans les grandes entreprises ou les organismes importants. Elles ont l'impression qu'elles vont poursuivre le développement de leurs carrières.

Un deuxième indice de la satisfaction au travail vient d'une question que nous avons posée sur les facteurs auxquels les répondantes accordaient le plus et le moins d'importance (Tableau 2). Parmi la liste des facteurs, il y en avait certains qui étaient liés au travail et d'autres qui avaient trait à d'autres dimensions de la vie. Le facteur qui est considéré comme le plus important pour ces femmes gestionnaires est l'intérêt du travail. La prédominance de cette réponse est claire. Pour illustrer cette conclusion, 39 % des répondantes ont dit que l'intérêt du travail était le facteur le plus important, la deuxième réponse pour ce qui est de la fréquence a été mentionnée par seulement 19% des personnes et, de surcroît, seulement une personne a mentionné ce facteur comme le moins important. En fait, 64% de toutes les répondantes ont dit que l'intérêt du travail était soit le facteur le plus important, soit le deuxième en importance.

Cette question était aussi intéressante parce qu'elle nous permettait de voir les combinaisons qui étaient valorisées par les femmes. La combinaison qui est revenue le plus souvent est l'intérêt du travail

Tableau 1
Futur cheminement de carrière

Futur cheminement de carrière	Nombre	%
Vertical	85	39,7
Developpement	49	22,9
Stable	42	19,6
Descendant	1	0,5
Réorientation	8	3,7
Retraite	8	3,7
Pas de plan	16	7,5
Choix à faire	5	2,3
	214	99,9

Tableau 2
Les facteurs les plus importants

Facteurs les plus importants	Premier choix nombre	%	Deuxième choix nombre	%
Revenu	13	6,1	15	7,0
Expérience	12	5,6	22	10,3
Ambiance	16	7,5	16	7,5
Temps-famille	41	19,2	31	14,5
Formation	5	2,3	5	2,3
Niveau de responsabilité	21	9,8	33	15,4
Sécurité d'emploi	3	1,4	7	3,3
Loisirs	3	1,4	5	2,3
Promotion	6	2,8	4	1,9
Intérêt de travail	85	39,7	52	24,3
Temps-amies	0	0,0	9	4,2
Plan de carrière	9	4,2	15	7,0
	214	100,0	214	100,0

et le temps consacré à la famille. Cette réponse indique que ces femmes recherchent une multidimensionnalité dans leur vie. Elles veulent équilibrer leur travail avec la vie hors travail. Le travail est extrêmement important mais il n'est pas tout dans la vie. Cette conclusion aurait été plus forte si dans notre formulation, les termes « temps consacré à la famille » avaient inclus les célibataires, car celles-ci avaient l'impression que cette réponse ne les touchait pas. Si nous avions formulé la réponse d'une façon plus globale pour référer à la sphère de la vie hors travail, les réponses auraient été, sans doute, encore plus fortes.

Finalement, nous avons demandé aux répondantes si elles consi-déraient que leur cheminement de carrière avait été pleinement satisfaisant, satisfaisant ou peu satisfaisant. Plus de la moitié, 110 sur 214, ont dit être pleinement satisfaites et presque autant, 92, s'es-timent satisfaites. Ces réponses confirment le portrait d'un groupe qui trouve son travail intéressant, qui veut poursuivre le dévelop-pement de sa carrière et qui croit en ce développement.

Comment peut-on expliquer cette situation? Nous allons tenter de démontrer que nos répondantes sont satisfaites parce qu'elles ne sont pas obligées de choisir une seule définition d'elles-mêmes, elles peuvent combiner différents aspects des rôles sociaux. Il nous semble que la capacité de concilier différentes définitions de soi est l'une des explications. Nous voulons voir les différentes formes de con-ciliation entre le travail et différentes dimensions de la vie hors travail, et aussi entre les exigences du travail et leur perception de leur situation de femme.

Pour illustrer la compatibilité entre le travail et la vie hors travail, nous allons nous baser sur un certain nombre d'indices. Première-ment, sur le plan concret, l'horaire de travail n'est pas incompatible avec la vie hors travail (Tableau 3). Par exemple, le nombre d'heures travaillées par semaine indique que le travail, quoique lourd, n'en-vahit pas la totalité de la vie. Presque la moitié des femmes disent travailler entre 40 et 49 heures par semaine (104 sur 214), ce qui représente une bonne semaine de travail, mais non pas un horaire empêchant toute autre forme d'activité. Environ 10% des répon-dantes estiment travailler plus de 60 heures, mais un nombre égal consacre entre 35 et 39 heures par semaine au travail. La plupart des répondantes ont un rythme de travail assez régulier, car presque les deux tiers disent quitter le travail plus ou moins à la même heure tous les jours. Et quoique la grande majorité doivent voyager pour le travail (seulement 30 personnes ont répondu jamais), la majorité de celles qui voyagent ont dit qu'elles planifient elles-mêmes leurs déplacements, profitant ainsi d'une marge de manoeuvre impor-tante. En fait, elles ont une certaine capacité pour organiser leur propre horaire de travail et peuvent donc organiser les liens entre le travail et la vie hors travail.

Un deuxième indice est que, pour beaucoup de nos répondantes, les activités sociales liées au travail ne sont pas considérées comme nécessaires pour réussir leur carrière. Le stéréotype des gestion-naires prises dans une gamme d'activités sociales absolument néces-saires à la réussite de leur carrière n'est pas le modèle adopté pour une partie importante de notre échantillon. Pour les répondantes, le travail se fait essentiellement dans les heures de travail et n'ac-

Tableau 3
Heures de travail par semaine

Heures de travail par semaine	Nombre	%
Moins de 35	1	0,5
35 à 39	25	11,7
40 à 49	104	48,6
50 à 59	59	27,6
60 et plus	25	11,7
	214	100,1

capare pas l'ensemble de la vie sociale. En fait, 33,6% des répondantes ont dit que les activités sociales étaient nécessaires pour leur carrière tandis que 33,26% exprimaient l'opposé. Un autre groupe de 28,5% les ont qualifiées d'utiles, mais non de nécessaires. De fait, elles déclarent passer peu de temps à ces activités sociales (Tableau 4). La majorité des répondantes ont dit consacrer moins de trois heures par mois à des activités sociales reliées au travail, seulement 8% des répondantes passant plus de 15 heures par mois à de telles activités. De plus, les gestionnaires vivant en couple accordent très peu de temps aux activités sociales liées au travail de leur conjoint. Seulement 15% des répondantes disent consacrer plus de trois heures par mois à ces activités. Leur travail ne semble donc pas envahi par un ensemble d'activités sociales; il déborde les heures au bureau dans certains cas, mais pour la plupart de nos répondantes, ce débordement est limité.

La possibilité d'une vie hors travail est accrue par le fait que les femmes déclarent recevoir de l'aide pour les travaux domestiques. Nous avons demandé aux femmes combien d'heures elles consacraient aux tâches domestiques par semaine et combien d'heures étaient consacrées par leurs conjoints. Les réponses indiquent d'une part que la majorité des gestionnaires ne considèrent pas le partage des tâches comme un partage égal, mais d'autre part elles considèrent que leurs conjoints consacrent du temps aux tâches domestiques. En plus de l'aide des conjoints, il est clair que nos répondantes ne font pas beaucoup de tâches domestiques – 41% des répondantes disent en faire moins de 8 heures par semaine et 11%, moins de trois heures. Nous pouvons soutenir que nos réponses indiquent que le travail domestique n'accapare pas tout le temps libre de nos répondantes. Elles peuvent avoir d'autres activités que leur travail rémunéré et les tâches domestiques. Il faut tout de même ajouter que

Tableau 4
Mes activités sociales pour mon travail

Activités sociales pour travail	Nombre	%
Rien	38	17,8
Moins de 3 heures	73	34,1
3 à 7	55	25,7
8 à 14	31	14,5
15 à 21	11	5,1
22 et plus	6	2,8
	214	100,0

relativement peu de nos répondantes vivent avec de jeunes enfants, ce dont il faut tenir compte dans l'interprétation de ces résultats.

Enfin, nous leur avons demandé combien de temps elles accordaient à des activités de loisir. La réponse la plus fréquente se situe entre 8 et 14 heures par semaine (80 répondantes), tandis que 65 répondantes leur consacrent plus de 15 heures par semaine. À la question du type d'activités de loisir préféré, les réponses indiquent une grande variété d'activités. Les sports sont mentionnés par beaucoup ainsi que les concerts, le théâtre, la lecture ... L'interprétation est plus difficile, car comment peut-on évaluer le temps de loisir? Est-ce peu ou est-ce que cela indique une possibilité réelle de participer à d'autres activités que celles du travail et de la maison?

Nous n'avons toutefois pas posé de question ni sur le mode de gestion des différents éléments de la vie ou sur la satisfaction des répondantes à l'égard de ces modes de gestion. Aucune intentionnalité n'était exprimée dans les questions, et si nous avons posé des questions de fait concernant différents aspects de la vie de nos répondantes, surtout de leur vie au travail, nous établissons des liens entre ces réponses. Nous considérons que leur travail en tant que gestionnaire constitue une des raisons pour lesquelles nos répondantes sont si satisfaites de leur travail tout en notant qu'il n'empêche pas une certaine vie hors du travail.

Comme deuxième élément d'explication en ce qui concerne la satisfaction de nos répondantes à l'égard de leur travail, on peut considérer que leur emploi n'est pas incompatible avec leur identification comme femmes ou, plutôt, nos répondantes ne se sentent pas obligées d'oublier qu'elles sont des femmes pour réussir leur carrière. Nos répondantes sont conscientes de la situation des femmes sur le marché du travail, mais elles ont une interprétation de la réalité qui leur permet de se percevoir comme femmes et, en même temps, de rester optimistes quant à leurs chances de gravir les échelons du pouvoir. Elles croient à la solidarité des femmes, elles agissent en fonction de cette solidarité et les contraintes qu'elles considèrent comme les plus importantes pour contrer l'avancement des femmes gestionnaires sont des facteurs qui, selon elles, peuvent changer dans l'avenir ou sont déjà au moins partiellement modifiés.

Nos résultats indiquent que les femmes croient à la solidarité des femmes et qu'elles agissent concrètement en fonction de ces objectifs. Les réponses à trois questions illustrent cette dimension. Tout d'abord, la grande majorité de nos répondantes considèrent qu'il est très important (121 sur 214) ou important (67 sur 214) pour les femmes de s'appuyer entre elles (Tableau 5). Mais, plus concrète-ment, les femmes disent qu'elles agissent comme mentor pour d'au-tres femmes (Tableau 6). En fait, 40% des répondantes ont été mentor surtout pour des femmes, 37% pour des femmes et des hommes, 7% surtout pour des hommes. Un autre indice de la soli-darité entre femmes, est que 60% des répondantes ont, souvent ou parfois, donné un appui particulier à quelqu'une parce que c'était une femme (Tableau 7).

Les femmes restent très conscientes de leur position comme fem-mes, mais elles ont en général une impression de cette position qui leur permet de se projeter dans l'avenir avec un certain optimisme. Elles mesurent les obstacles, mais elles entrevoient aussi des méca-nismes facilitant le cheminement des femmes gestionnaires. Ainsi nous avons demandé aux femmes d'indiquer (dans une série de réponses possibles) ce qu'elles considéraient comme un obstacle ou un mécanisme facilitant. Les résultats globaux indiquent que les répondantes ont identifié plus d'obstacles que de mécanismes fa-cilitants, mais les résultats sont assez partagés pour quelques ré-ponses. Par exemple, dans le cas de la composition des comités de sélection, 33 gestionnaires perçoivent cet élément comme un obstacle important tandis que pour 34 d'entre elles, il est un mécanisme facilitant. Dans certains cas, les répondantes semblent avoir inter-prété les questions de façon très différente tandis que dans d'autres cas, ce sont les évaluations qui diffèrent. De toutes les réponses, un facteur ressort clairement comme un obstacle important, c'est celui du peu de femmes cadres qui sont gestionnaires dans leur propre organisme. L'obstacle principal est donc un élément qui peut se modifier dans un délai raisonnable quand ce n'est pas déjà mis en place. Ce phénomène est semblable aux réponses que nous avions obtenu dans une question ouverte pour mesurer si elles avaient dû faire face à d'autres obstacles au cours de leur carrière. Dans la

Tableau 5
Importance pour les femmes de s'appuyer

Importance	Nombre	%
Oui, très important	121	56,5
Oui, assez important	67	31,3
Non, pas très important	22	10,3
Non, pas du tout important	4	1,9
	214	100,0

Tableau 6
Mentor pour d'autres personnes

Réponse	Nombre	%
Non	32	15,0
Surtout femmes	87	40,7
Surtout hommes	16	7,5
Pour les deux	79	36,9
	214	100,1

Tableau 7
Appui particulier aux femmes

Réponse	Nombre	%
Oui, souvent	60	28,0
Oui, parfois	71	33,2
Non, jamais fait	42	19,6
Non, je m'y oppose	37	17,3
Si compétence	4	1,9
	214	100,0

plupart des cas, les obstacles mentionnés tiennent à des attitudes et très souvent les femmes ont ajouté que ces attitudes sont à même de changer, car s'il y a encore des hommes qui ne sont pas à l'aise avec les femmes gestionnaires, bon nombre d'entre eux sont devenus plus habiles à interagir avec des femmes. Pour la plupart des répondantes, les éléments qui entravent ou facilitent le cheminement de carrière des femmes, ainsi que leur conception de la solidarité entre les femmes impliquent que la « réussite » de la carrière de gestionnaire est possible sans oublier pour autant qu'elles sont des femmes.

BIBLIOGRAPHIE

Adler, Nancy J. and Dafna N. Izraeli, eds. 1988. *Women in Management Worldwide.*New York: M.E. Sharpe, Inc.

Aubert, Nicole 1982. *Le pouvoir usurpé.* Paris, Robert-Laffont.

Andrew, Caroline, Cécile Coderre et Ann Denis 1988a. « Women in Management, the Canadian Experience. » *Women in Management Worldwide:* New York: M.E. Sharpe, Inc. 250–64.

Armstrong, Pat and Hugh Armstrong 1984. *The Double Ghetto.* 2nd edition. Toronto: McClelland and Stewart.

David, Hélène 1986. *Femmes et emploi. Le défi de l'égalité.* Sillery (Québec): Presses de l'Université du Québec.

Gutek, Barbara and Laurie Larwood, eds. 1986. *Women's Career Development.* California: Sage Publications.

Harel-Giasson, Francine 1981. *Perception et actualisation des facteurs de promotion chez les femmes cadres des grandes entreprises québécoises francophones du secteur privé.* Thèse de doctorat. Montréal, HEC

Huppert-Laufer, Jacqueline 1982. *La féminité neutralisée? Les femmes cadres dans l'entreprise.* Paris, Flammarion.

Kanter, Rosabeth Moss 1977. *Men and Women of the Corporation.* New York: Basic Books.

Marshall, Judi 1984. *Women Managers. Travellers in a Male World,* Great Britain: John Wiley & Sons.

Symons, Gladys 1982. « La carrière! Un vécu au féminin. » *Gestion* (septembre).

GHYSLAINE SAVARIA

Femmes collaboratrices et plénitude

On retrouve partout au Canada environ 560 000 femmes collaboratrices qui exploitent avec leur mari une entreprise appartenant en tout ou en partie à ce dernier. Réalité encore peu connue il y a quelques années, le travail des collaboratrices est aujourd'hui de plus en plus valorisé de telle sorte que ces femmes s'acheminent désormais vers la plénitude. Dans les PME, les entreprises agricoles et les bureaux professionnels où elles évoluent, les femmes collaboratrices se perçoivent maintenant comme de réelles partenaires de leur mari. Pour plusieurs d'entre elles cependant, l'absence d'une rémunération adéquate vient ternir le tableau de la satisfaction au travail. Grâce à l'Association des femmes collaboratrices, elles gravissent les échelons de la reconnaissance de leur travail.

Women-in-Partnership and Fulfillment

In Canada, about 560,000 women in partnership with their husbands operate a business belonging in whole or in part to their spouses. Although this phenomenon was not well known a few years ago, the work of such women is becoming more and more valued, and these women are experiencing greater satisfaction. In the small and medium-businesses, agriculture, and professional offices where they work, women in partnership now see themselves as the true equals of their husbands. For many, however, the lack of adequate remuneration diminishes their satisfaction with work. Through the Association of Wives in Family Businesses, they are beginning to receive more recognition for their work.

C'est en travaillant à leur mieux-être et à celui de leur famille dans l'entreprise familiale, en essayant de réaliser l'équilibre épanouissant de femme, épouse et femme d'affaires, que les femmes collaboratrices sont en marche vers leur plénitude.

Cet exposé développera ce thème en essayant de répondre à trois questions:

- Qui sont ces femmes collaboratrices?
- Comment, dans leur vie quotidienne, s'acheminent-elles vers leur mieux-être?
- Quels sont les moyens qu'elles se donnent pour éliminer les obstacles à leur plénitude?

PROFIL DES FEMMES COLLABORATRICES

Mais qui sont donc ces femmes collaboratrices? Que font-elles? Où sont-elles? Précisons au départ que beaucoup de petites entreprises n'existeraient pas sans l'apport d'une conjointe collaboratrice. Pour ne citer que mon expérience personnelle, en 1965, mon mari, nouveau propriétaire d'une tout aussi nouvelle entreprise de transport, s'installait chaque matin au volant de notre unique camion tandis que je me postais au téléphone pour prendre les commandes des clients et préparer les soumissions. Vingt ans plus tard, notre compagnie compte une dizaine de camions et 15 employées. Je suis consciente qu'à deux, on est arrivé plus vite à donner de l'expansion à notre entreprise et que ma participation a été déterminante.

Si l'expression « femme collaboratrice » est nouvelle, la réalité, elle, existe depuis toujours. Votre grand-mère et la mienne étaient probablement de ces femmes qui consacraient de longues heures au travail de la ferme ou à la tenue du commerce.

Au Canada, on compte 560 000 femmes collaboratrices. On les retrouve dans l'entreprise agricole, dans les petites entreprises commerciales et dans les bureaux professionnels; dans ces entreprises qui appartiennent en tout ou en partie à leur mari, en partie signifiant que l'associée du mari peut être sa femme ou une autre.

Pour en tracer plus précisément le profil, reportons-nous à l'enquête menée au Québec en 1984 par Ruth Rose-Lizée, professeure de sciences économiques à l'Université du Québec à Montréal. Celle-ci démontre que ces femmes ont en moyenne 40 ans, 3 enfants, 18 ans de mariage et travaillent depuis 11 ans dans l'entreprise de leur conjoint.

Parmi les femmes interrogées, 57% ont un niveau d'études secondaires, 22% post-secondaires. Leur statut légal: 6% sont actionnaires, 5% copropriétaires, 1,6% associées. Elles travaillent 40 heures par semaine et beaucoup plus durant certaines saisons ou périodes de pointe. Moins de 40% reçoivent un salaire, dont la moyenne hebdomadaire est de $168, ce montant étant souvent absorbé par les besoins de la famille.

Il est important de mentionner que 8 sur 10 de ces femmes travaillant avec leur mari dans l'entreprise familiale n'ont pas de statut légal en fonction du droit commercial. Si la reconnaissance légale et financière du travail des femmes est loin d'être uniforme, les niveaux de collaboration entre conjoint et conjointe sont eux aussi très différents d'une entreprise à l'autre. Les tâches accomplies au sein de leur entreprise en témoignent explicitement. En effet, parmi les femmes consultées, 40,1% font la comptabilité et la tenue de livres, 30% s'occupent de la supervision du personnel, 28,1% participent au travail de la ferme, tandis que 19.8% remplissent les fonctions de secrétaire. Quant aux autres, elles sont réceptionnistes ou téléphonistes, s'occupent des ventes, de l'administration, etc.

DANS LEUR VIE QUOTIDIENNE, LES FEMMES COLLABORATRICES S'ACHEMINENT VERS LEUR MIEUX-ÊTRE

Ces femmes sont contentes de leur travail; elles y trouvent satisfaction et épanouissement. Si les collaboratrices ont choisi de travailler avec leur mari, c'est pour des raisons affectives et économiques communes. Ce qui les motive, c'est qu'elles aiment travailler avec leur mari et que ce partenariat leur permet très souvent de bien faire démarrer l'entreprise familiale. En travaillant pour celle-ci, elles considèrent qu'elles sont plus libres qu'ailleurs, elles peuvent développer leurs capacités et faire preuve de plus d'initiative tout en garantissant aux leurs et en se garantissant à elles-mêmes une meilleure qualité de vie au travail. Ainsi, reconnaissent-elles qu'elles peuvent s'épanouir personnellement en tant que femmes et concilier l'éducation de leurs enfants et une vie familiale harmonieuse.

Soulignons bien que si ces femmes ont choisi d'être collaboratrices, c'est parce que ce travail leur plaît et non pas parce que c'était leur « devoir de femme ».

Ces femmes veulent réussir en amour et en affaires. Les femmes des jeunes couples pour qui la collaboration se réalise de plus en plus au début du mariage, à tout le moins dès la création de l'entreprise, ou celles des plus vieux couples, pour qui elle se fait en cours de route, le disent elles-mêmes: le fonctionnement du couple a une importance primordiale dans la relation de travail. Si le couple va, tout va. Il n'est pas rare que la bonne entente conjugale tienne lieu d'entente commerciale. C'est souvent le cas des femmes non salariées, qui travailleront sans toucher de salaire pour le bénéfice de l'entreprise familiale. Heureusement que dans bien des cas, cette situation sera corrigée quand la vitalité de l'entreprise sera garantie ou quand les propriétaires conjoints ne tiendront pas à maintenir indûment l'inégalité de cette situation.

Peu importe à quel moment commence la collaboration, un point est commun à toutes ces femmes: elles investissent temps, argent, énergie et souvent tout ce qu'elles sont pour la réussite de leur entreprise familiale. Elles ont en même temps le sentiment que ce faisant, elles participent aussi à la réussite de leur vie de couple.

On peut dire aussi que d'une façon générale, les collaboratrices jouissent d'une responsabilité et d'un pouvoir significatif au sein de l'entreprise. Leurs maris les consultent avant de prendre les décisions importantes, financières ou autres, et tiennent compte de leur opinion même quand elle ne correspond pas à la leur. C'est pourquoi elles pensent que l'entreprise aurait de la difficulté à fonctionner sans elles.

Ainsi, on peut prendre conscience du véritable rôle de partenaire que jouent, à des degrés divers, les femmes collaboratrices et ce, notamment, à travers trois fonctions qu'elles exercent. Voyons sommairement en quoi consistent ces fonctions.

D'abord n'oublions pas que les collaboratrices évoluent généralement dans des entreprises de petite taille qui requièrent, pour leur prospérité, un haut niveau d'entreprenariat. Comme les collaboratrices sont directement concernées par les hauts et les bas de leur commerce, de leur exploitation agricole, du professionnel qu'elles assistent ou autres, on peut s'attendre à ce qu'elles prennent aussi part au défi concurrentiel de l'entreprise.

Les entrepreneures, avant tout, ont la responsabilité de prendre toutes les décisions concernant l'entreprise. D'après l'enquête, on constate que 86,6% des femmes collaboratrices prennent seules des décisions dans l'entreprise familiale, et que 80,2% d'entre elles ont l'impression de participer à part entière aux efforts de l'entreprise.

Les entrepreneures, ce sont aussi celles qui prennent l'initiative de combiner les ressources naturelles, le capital et le travail, afin de produire des biens et des services. Or, dans l'enquête citée auparavant, 9 répondantes sur 10 affirment participer régulièrement aux décisions sur les grosses dépenses tandis que 3 sur 10 disent superviser des employés-es dans l'entreprise.

Il est donc juste d'affirmer que les collaboratrices, en tant que partenaires entrepreneures, fournissent un effort complémentaire à celui de leur mari pour assurer le développement de l'entreprise familiale.

Le niveau de complémentarité variera selon les fonctions des collaboratrices dans l'entreprise ainsi que selon la nature de celle-ci (exploitation agricole, PME, secteur professionnel), mais dans tous les cas, les femmes collaboratrices demeurent de véritables partenaires de leur conjoint dans une démarche de croissance de l'entreprise.

Les collaboratrices sont aussi *des femmes d'affaires* puisqu'elles exercent un ensemble cohérent d'activités industrielles, agricoles, commerciales ou financières pour leur propre compte et celui de leur mari. Avec eux, elles ont à coeur la réussite de l'entreprise.

C'est à travers les diverses fonctions qu'elles exercent au sein de l'entreprise que l'on peut mieux constater qu'elles agissent comme femmes d'affaires.

Elles prennent ou influencent des décisions qui touchent le roulement ou l'avenir de l'entreprise. Cette étape est souvent précédée d'une négociation avec leur mari.

Elles travaillent à optimiser les ressources humaines pour offrir un meilleur produit ou un meilleur service et pour maintenir ou augmenter la rentabilité de l'entreprise. Elles feront la promotion de celle-ci; on les retrouvera souvent aux relations publiques. D'une façon générale, comme femmes d'affaires, partenaires de leur conjoint, elles participent à la bonne marche de l'entreprise familiale et on peut dire que leur rôle est de première importance.

Les fonctions d'affaires exercées par les collaboratrices sont sans doute celles qui contribuent le plus au développement de l'entreprise, surtout lorsqu'elles s'étendent sur plusieurs années, faisant ainsi bénéficier l'entreprise d'une expérience, d'une expertise et de relations irremplaçables. L'enquête précitée souligne à ce sujet que 52,5% des femmes collaboratrices avaient déjà, en 1984, investi plus de 10 ans de travail dans l'entreprise familiale et que même jusqu'à 22,1% avaient à leur actif plus de 20 ans de loyaux services!!! Voyons là une indication significative du rôle des collaboratrices dans le maintien et l'expansion de l'entreprise.

Il nous faut reconnaître aussi aux collaboratrices, leur rôle de *gestionnaires*.

À ce titre, notre précieuse enquête nous révèle que 7,5% d'entre elles font précisément un travail d'administration alors que 44,7% s'occupent de comptabilité et de tenue de livres dans l'entreprise familiale.

On peut donc affirmer que plus de la moitié des femmes collaboratrices sont concernées par des activités de gestion et que la plupart du temps, c'est au niveau des ressources financières que s'exerce la prise de décision.

Pour ce qui est de la gestion des ressources humaines, on a déjà vu que 3 femmes sur 10 supervisent le travail d'employés-es. On sait aussi que le quart d'entre elles sont responsables du travail de plus de cinq employés-es, ce qui équivaut presque à de la gestion de personnel à plein temps.

En se préoccupant avec leur mari d'une saine administration des ressources humaines et financières, on peut reconnaître que les femmes collaboratrices agissent en gestionnaires dans l'entreprise familiale.

Cette implication comme partenaires-entrepreneures, femmes d'affaires et gestionnaires variera selon le contexte où se vit le partenariat et le type d'entreprise économique concerné, bien entendu. Mais nous pouvons affirmer qu'à des degrés divers, les femmes collaboratrices sont l'une et l'autre à la fois ou tour à tour.

C'est à travers toutes ces activités au sein de l'entreprise qu'elles développent compétence, sens de l'organisation, de la gestion, esprit d'analyse, capacité de prendre des décisions, goût du risque. Par le fait qu'elles oeuvrent dans une entreprise familiale comme partenaire du conjoint, elles ont l'occasion de redécouvrir et d'exploiter leurs qualités de négociatrices, de communicatrices, leur sens de l'intuition, de la prospective et leurs aptitudes à créer les conditions pour une meilleure qualité de vie au travail autant que dans la famille.

Comme on peut le constater, c'est dans leur quotidien que ces femmes cheminent, s'affirment, prennent conscience de ce qu'elles sont, de ce qu'elles veulent vivre et, ce faisant, elles vont de plus en plus vers la réalisation d'elles-mêmes, de leur autonomie, de leur mieux-être et par là, de leur plénitude.

Mais malgré tout, dans ce qu'elles veulent vivre, il y a des ombres au tableau. À cette satisfaction du travail dans l'entreprise, une insatisfaction persiste. Ces femmes qui investissent temps, énergie et argent dans l'entreprise familiale sont encore des travailleuses invisibles. Elles n'ont pas de statut comme tel et, bien souvent, elles n'apparaissent pas sur la liste de paye de l'entreprise et ne figurent pas dans les statistiques de l'emploi. Une collaboratrice sur deux n'est ni protégée par le droit commercial, ni en vertu du contrat de mariage. Que surviennent la rupture de l'union, le décès du mari ou la vente de l'entreprise et plusieurs se retrouveront sans gagne-pain et sans rétribution pour les années de travail consacrées à l'entreprise. On n'a qu'à se rappeler le cas de Rosa Becker, cette femme qui s'est suicidée parce qu'elle n'avait pas obtenu justice, des années après avoir fait reconnaître son travail par les tribunaux. Bien d'autres n'ont pas fait la manchette des journaux.

L'ASSOCIATION DES FEMMES COLLABORATRICES : UN MOYEN POUR ATTEINDRE LEUR MIEUX-ÊTRE

Depuis le 29 mars 1980, l'Association des femmes collaboratrices oeuvre pour que le travail de ces femmes soit reconnu sur le plan légal, fiscal et social. Il est temps qu'on prenne conscience de l'apport des collaboratrices à l'entreprise et à la société. Lors de l'enquête de 1984, on estimait à 9 milliards de dollars leur contribution à l'économie canadienne, ce qui constituait environ 3% du revenu national net, revenu qui vient d'une source gardée « invisible ».

Parce que la part de travail apportée par les collaboratrices a une valeur certaine et non évaluée, ne permettant pas à l'entreprise d'établir ses coûts réels d'exploitation.

Parce que la part de travail fournie par la salariée est une activité mesurable. Si ce travail était exercé dans une autre entreprise, il serait évalué selon les normes et rémunéré comme tel, permettant l'accès aux mesures fiscales pour l'entreprise, et aux avantages sociaux et professionnels pour les collaboratrices.

Parce que la part de travail investie dans l'administration, la gestion et la production demande expérience et compétence.

Parce que ce travail doit assurer la sécurité et l'autonomie financière de celle et celui qui y participent: la femme et l'homme qui collaborent.

Des collaboratrices se sont regroupées pour faire connaître sur le plan économique la valeur distincte de leur travail au sein de l'entreprise familiale et revendiquer la déclaration d'un statut de femme collaboratrice. L'Association des femmes collaboratrices travaille, à l'échelle du Canada,

à sensibiliser la population en général et les différents organismes publics aux problèmes de la collaboratrice; à chercher des solutions appropriées aux différentes situations vécues; à permettre aux femmes, membres de l'Association, de pousser la réflexion sur leur situation personnelle à l'intérieur du couple et de la famille.

Cette association veut en même temps fournir à ces femmes une formation adéquate susceptible d'améliorer la qualité de leur travail au sein de l'entreprise familiale.

À ces situations qu'elles vivaient isolément, elles opposent, en se regroupant, la compréhension, le soutien et la solidarité dans la poursuite d'un objectif commun. Le mouvement devient pour elles l'instrument qui leur permettra d'atteindre leur mieux-être. Cette poursuite dans l'acquisition des droits et avantages réclamés pour les collaboratrices accroît leur motivation au travail dans l'entreprise, les stimule à exploiter tout leur potentiel et les conduit inévitablement vers l'atteinte de leur plénitude, c'est-à-dire de leur réalisation complète comme femmes et travailleuses reconnues.

CONCLUSION

Tant que cette reconnaissance n'est pas obtenue, cette démarche vers la plénitude s'accomplit d'abord par chacune, dans sa réalité quotidienne. Puis collectivement, regroupées au sein de l'Association des femmes collaboratrices elles travaillent à ce que cette plénitude devienne un espoir pour toutes, c'est-à-dire que ces femmes voient, dans un avenir rapproché, leur valeur reconnue sur le plan légal et social, et cela d'un océan à l'autre.

BIBLIOGRAPHIE

Rose-Lizée, Ruth (1985). *Portrait des femmes collaboratrices du Québec/1984.* St-Lambert: Association des femmes collaboratrices.

GLORIA R. GELLER

Maintaining Separate Spheres: Women's Efforts to Enter Non-traditional Jobs – A Pilot Study of Women Working in Corrections in Saskatchewan[1]

A pilot study of ten women working as corrections workers in male institutions was undertaken in order to explore the experiences of women in this non-traditional job. Data gathered in interviews included; information about the positions the women hold in correctional institutions, how women are treated, obstacles they encounter, experiences of harassment, how they deal with security issues and violence, the nature of the stresses experienced and how they deal with these stresses. For some women the experience has been a difficult one and the price they pay is high. Some of the women believe they have overcome many of the obstacles they have faced and have achieved some level of acceptance within the field of corrections.

Le maintien de sphères séparées:
les efforts des femmes pour occuper des emplois non traditionnels –
une étude pilote sur les femmes oeuvrant dans
les services correctionnels en Saskatchewan

Une étude pilote sur dix femmes travaillant dans des établissements correctionnels pour hommes a été entreprise afin d'examiner les expériences vécues par les femmes occupant ces emplois non traditionnels. Les entrevues ont permis de recueillir des renseignements notamment sur les postes que les femmes occupent dans les établissements correctionnels, le traitement dont elles font l'objet, les obstacles qu'elles doivent surmonter, leurs expériences en matière de harcèlement, comment elles abordent les questions de sécurité et la violence, la nature des stress qu'elles connaissent et comment elles les surmontent. Pour certaines femmes, l'expérience a été difficile, et le prix à payer élevé. Certaines croient avoir surmonté les obstacles auxquels elles étaient confrontées, et avoir réussi à obtenir une certaine reconnaissance dans le domaine des services correctionnels.

INTRODUCTION

Women's role within patriarchal culture has been defined as a nurturing or expressive one, and many predominantly female jobs appear to be extensions of their roles in the family. There has been differentiation between men's and women's tasks in jobs dealing with people in such fields as medicine, where nursing is largely (in North America) a female job and doctoring a male job. A number of other "people-oriented" jobs are viewed as men's jobs; women have not been permitted entry because of concern about their physical strength and the dangers these jobs pose. In particular, policing and correctional work have been off-limits to women until recently, except for very specific areas, usually those related to work with young people, with women, or both.

Specific issues raised in respect to the introduction of women working in male correctional institutions have led to the exclusion of women from certain jobs in corrections. Questions concerning women's ability to deal with violence are frequently raised. The system has tended to place women in specific jobs which are considered more appropriate for them. In addition, women may be given preferential treatment or offered protection which in the long run could act as detriments to them if they have not adequately learned to take care of themselves (Baunach 1982). The concerns most frequently expressed are related to their being alone on the tiers of a prison and their vulnerability to physical attack and sexual assault.

Interestingly, the literature on policing and corrections does not actually find that women are more vulnerable or experience greater difficulty than men, but previous research shows that men in the system have great difficulty with women's involvement in the work and believe women lack the ability to handle violent situations (Linden and Minch 1982; Baunach 1982; Wilson 1982; Flynn 1982). Research findings, on the other hand, tend to show that women deal adequately with violent situations and that other skills, including tact, diplomacy, competence, and certain personality characteristics, are often more useful than sheer brawn in handling such situations (Linden and Minch 1982; Flynn 1982; Kissel and Katsampes 1980). In fact, the literature shows that women may have a "softening" effect in prisons. Women have been responsible for the de-escalation of violent or potentially violent situations.

The second major rationale for limiting women's involvement in correctional institutions is the issue of inmates' rights to privacy. The need to guard against the intrusion upon prisoners' rights is used to justify keeping women out of the system or away from certain jobs in the institution. Inmates in the United States have brought suits claiming that their rights to privacy have been violated (Feinman 1980). Reforms which can reconcile employing women in the system with inmate rights are quite feasible. Feinman (1980, 56) reports that California fully integrated women into the state correctional system in 1974. As a general rule, women officers in California do not do skin searches of male inmates, nor do men skin-search female inmates. Screens have been put up in shower and toilet facilities, leaving only the upper body visible and windows have been fogged so that only outlines of bodies can be seen. Inmates have not complained and officers have not encountered insoluble difficulties. A further benefit has been that male officers show more respect for inmates' privacy.

Women as workers are rejected in the criminal justice system, in policing and corrections, not by the inmates or offenders they deal with but by their co-workers (Linden and Minch 1982; Kissel and Katsampes 1980). Studies of community responses toward women police officers indicate a favourable reaction (Linden and Minch 1982). It is less clear whether administrators are responding positively. Below, a study conducted among women correctional workers in Saskatchewan explores these and other issues more fully.

PILOT STUDY: WOMEN WORKING IN CORRECTIONS IN SASKATCHEWAN

Marie Sakowski (1985–86, 52–3) describes the situation of three of the first women in Canada to be hired as correctional officers in federal male penitentiaries. She states that the women were given special but subordinate status. They were subjected to intense scrutiny by the security department, as compared to male corrections workers. The most significant factor in their subordination was, according to Sakowski, the harassment and intense hostility they experienced from their male colleagues who appeared to be trying to push the women out of the institution.

The picture Sakowski paints is a grim one. While it is not surprising that there may be initial problems in integrating women into occupations previously defined as male, after five years one would expect that the women would feel comfortable in their jobs. According to Sakowski's study, this was not the case.

To explore women's experiences in corrections further, a pilot study was undertaken in Saskatchewan to examine the situation of women corrections workers in both provincial and federal male institutions.

Taped interviews were conducted with ten women working in three correctional institutions in Saskatchewan – two provincial institutions and one federal penitentiary. The data are summarized in three parts:

Part A: Data about the respondents, the positions they hold, adjustments they have made for the job, what they like and dislike about their jobs.

Part B: Experiences working in corrections, how women are treated, obstacles encountered, harassment, working relationships, responses of family and friends and finally, women's experiences with security and violence on the job.

Part C: Stress experienced and how they deal with stress, hostility and harassment.

A   *The Respondents*

The positions held by the ten women who were interviewed include corrections worker, security officer, recreation officer, program counsellor, and case management officer. The women had worked in corrections between eight months and eight years. All but one were employed on a full-time basis. The employment background of the women is varied. Some had worked in low-paying, relatively unskilled jobs in sales, as labourers, or in store security, while others had completed university degrees and had been employed in human service positions, recreation, and counselling. For several women, corrections work was their first job after completing their schooling. Some women had studied criminology or related disciplines and entered corrections as a career choice.

We should make a clear distinction between those for whom the position represents a secure, well-paying job and those who had a university education and were seeking a career. The women working for the federal corrections system were more likely to have higher qualifications than those working in provincial institutions.

In response to a question about what they like and dislike in their jobs, the women identified more that they liked than that they disliked. In discussing their likes, the women particularly indicated the challenges and variety the job offered. Several mentioned that they liked working with inmates and others enjoyed working with co-workers. Several found working conditions to be positive and mentioned the fact that the salary was good. A couple of examples follow:

I think I use most of my capabilities almost every day. I would exhaust my repertoire of abilities every day and find some that I don't know I had. The expansion of yourself was phenomenal, how much you could do in a short while.

It is a challenge every day because everything is different. There is never any book answer to anything. You have to handle every situation differently which brings a challenge within yourself.

In answer to what they dislike, some noted that the job was conducive to high rates of burnout. Some complained about the disrupting effects of shift work. One was critical of her superiors and the attitudes of male co-workers toward women corrections workers. One complained of sexual harassment from inmates.

The respondents were asked about the adjustments they made to the job. The responses ranged widely from very few to very major behavioural and attitudinal changes. For some the cost has been high while for others it has been minimal. Some of the major adjustments the women have had to make are discussed below.

One woman described her experience in quite graphic terms:

I think it would be the kind of adjustment that you would make if you were living and working on the moon. Everybody you knew before who has never been to the moon doesn't know what you are talking about and can't really empathize with what is happening.

One woman discussed the adjustments required to work with prisoners:

You have to get used to working with people in a setting in which they don't want to be. These people don't want to be there so you have to get used to dealing with them in a way so that you can be diplomatic and still try to get them to do what it is you're supposed to be doing and what it is you want them to do. Lots of times the first thing that they do if you ask them to do something, they'll say "no" just because they don't want to be there and they're going to make life miserable for everybody.

B   Women as Correctional Workers

The women were asked whether women, when they start to work in corrections, are treated differently than men. Most of the women stated that they do receive different treatment from men in the same position. The women felt they had to prove themselves more than men usually do and that they were watched more closely. A woman who does not do well on the job is seen as representative of *all* women, whereas it would be thought absurd to blame all men if one did not perform well. Below are examples of their comments:

I certainly was treated differently, I was pretty much told that I wasn't welcome, that it was a field for men and they didn't really think I needed to be there.

These fellows don't relate to women. The staff really are used to the women they know, their mothers, their sisters, their wives, who may or may not work outside the home. She has children and her job is mainly to cater to them. Most of the men are really very chauvinistic. Their women have a place which is under their wing and they're very protective. They don't quite know what to think of you. Where do they place you in their memory bank as to what a woman should be?

In response to a question about the obstacles they encountered as women working in corrections, most stated that many male co-workers do not want women working with them. Some women stated that there were no opportunities for promotion. Several believed that the Human Rights exemption which prevents women from conducting skin frisks on male inmates is an obstacle in their work.

Women were asked whether they received preferential treatment within the system, whether they were protected by their male co-workers or supervisory staff, and whether women were able to deal with violence and security situations. The women denied that they received any preferential treatment and indeed stated that they were seriously penalized because they could not work in all parts of the institution.

Some women felt that their male co-workers thought that they were protecting the women, but the women were resentful at being prevented from participating in tense or violent situations. They were all confident in their abilty to do correctional work.

The women also indicated that men and women corrections workers may respond differently in a potential confrontation with an inmate. They stated that if a male correctional worker and an inmate meet in a confrontation, the inmate cannot back down without losing face, so the situation escalates. The women believe this is less likely to happen with a woman corrections worker. A woman may be able to walk into a situation and defuse it in cases where a male worker cannot.

One of the responses to questions of preferential treatment and protection follows:

In their minds it's protection, but in our minds we're being slighted. We can do the job. Say a fellow's acting out and has to be shackled and moved to a more secure area. A woman can walk beside a shackled man as easily as a man. It makes us look bad to put us in an isolated area and use a man to do something we could do.

In response to whether women can and should handle violent situations, all were adamant that they should and could, as their responses show:

I think they can handle security ... they are definitely not as strong as a man, but when we go on course we are taught the different restraints and it has got nothing to do with strength. It's technique. If you put a hold on right it doesn't matter how strong you are as long as you have it on right. So as long as they are trained the same way, no problem.

I've seen men walk into a situation and just call them every name in the book and then the shit hits the fan. I'm sure it has happened that female security staff have insulted male inmates but I've never heard it.

Another woman stated:

An inmate thanked me for not hurting him when we had him on the floor. He was subdued. I felt no reason to continue hurting him by holding his leg at the time. He laughed afterwards, not that day, but some time afterwards, he said "Thank you, you were the only one that didn't hurt me. I wasn't moving and they continued to hurt me."

The women had been involved in potentially dangerous and violent situations and felt they were capable of handling them. Indeed, at times they were able to defuse the situation, yet they were not trusted by their male co-workers and supervisors to respond to such situations. Clearly, women may have something important to teach men about responding in ways that defuse rather than escalate potentially dangerous situations.

The women were asked about their relationships with inmates, co-workers and supervisors. Most of the women indicated that they now felt accepted but almost all have experienced considerable difficulty gaining acceptance. The major problem they confronted in their working relationships has been with their male co-workers. This situation is common for women entering any type of non-traditional work. Once women are hired in such jobs they often confront considerable hostility and harassment by male counterparts

An indication of the women's tenuous position in the field of corrections can be seen by the remarks of the following respondent. Her remarks suggest that she cannot relax, and that another woman's actions could raise questions about her own position. It is very unlikely that a man in her position would make the following remarks about other men.

I'd like to see more women in corrections but it scares me because once you've worked really hard to get your own position, I resent the dipsy females that come in and bring up all the old issues I've already had to deal with. There's always that fear when new women start that they're going to do something that's going to bring the public eye or the internal eye upon women. We all suffer if one screws up.

One of the women discussed the fact that women who were introduced into the correctional system in Saskatchewan when new correctional centres (known as living units) were opened were put into a double bind. Because they were women, it was expected that they would interact with inmates in a very different manner from male corrections workers. The results of this situation caused a great deal of resentment from male corrections workers and problems for the women. She explained:

When we first opened it was so new having women in a closed setting like a living unit. I know that they figured it would just be so good because these fellows wouldn't swear as much because there's a woman around, and they would keep themselves tidier, they would comb their hair and brush their teeth and just to have a woman here would be like having a woman in the home or something like that. And that's how we were viewed. Whereas now I think, at least the women who have been here since the place opened, are being seen a little differently. We're capable. We're competent. We can be helpful in a situation where there's perhaps violence or someone is injured. We're not just fixtures that facilitate a homey atmosphere. We do something too. We have brains.

While learning the job was difficult it is also apparent from the following that women were set up for serious problems with co-workers and inmates because of the sexist assumptions of the administration:

When I first started my job it was very hard because I was the biggest shoulder to cry on. We were encouraged to do as much for them as we could. If they had a special hobby that they enjoyed, drawing, painting, whatever, we were encouraged to bring them things that were hard for them to get. We were encouraged to bake cookies. They led us totally astray when we first started here. Bring hominess into the unit at Christmas time, make popcorn balls and peanut brittle, and we did all this stuff with management's okay.

The first half of the five and one-half years I was here were pretty bad. We had an incident where one of the inmates had this idea that he was totally in love with one of the female staff. She was his woman. When he moved to a more secure area he told everyone that she slept with him on the night shift in his room. The staff precipitated that rumour which made it very difficult.

The male staff resented the time the female staff spent with inmates. That's what we were told to do when we started. You played cards with them. You talked to them. You watched TV with them. You had your meals with them. That's your job, to be there and become aware of how they think and feel and if they're having any problems, if they're suicidal, if they're having family problems. Normalize them in a family setting.

You have management saying, spend as much time with inmates as possible when you're on duty. You have the male staff sitting in the office, yakking, drinking coffee. So I would go in there, and the dirty jokes, the foul language, I would get to the point that I'd rather be with the inmates.

I'm getting more respect from the inmates. That has changed, I got very, very hard, very hard shelled. I also got used to the foul language and the innuendos. I take nothing personally. I give nothing personally. There's still a little softness in there somewhere but it very seldom comes out.

This woman was forced to change because of the harassment she experienced and the misinterpretation of her actions by inmates and male staff members. By asking women to do the job differently *because* they were women, management put them in an extremely difficult position. Management's views and expectations of women were, at this point, clearly very stereotyped.

The women's actions are frequently interpreted not only by management but also by staff and inmates in a stereotyped, sexualized manner. Women are therefore not responded to as people but as sexual beings. In the case just cited, the system viewed "normalization" in terms of stereotyped roles for the women who would bring cookies, talk to the inmates, and behave as nurturers rather than as typical corrections workers. This caused a great deal of difficulty between men and women corrections workers. Sexual comments and innuendos were often used by inmates and workers, and the women became immune to the continuous harassment and sexualizing of the women trying to work in a difficult situation.

When the women are victimized by sexual harassment, they are very careful not to upset their harasser so as not to cause themselves any further problems. As women and as workers, they walk a very fine line, feeling they have to exercise a great deal of caution in order to gain the acceptance of their co-workers and supervisors in a field where they hold very tenuous positions.

Women who try to break some of the limitations placed on them through social proscriptions may lack social supports for what they are seeking to do. They are likely to have to deal with negative, or at best neutral, responses to their efforts. Women seeking to enter non-traditional jobs may face negative responses from those whom they may otherwise count on for support, family members and friends.

If they lack such supports, then the few women with whom they work will be the support system they need in order to carry on in difficult circumstances. A major barrier for women in non-traditional jobs is their experience of isolation.

The women in this study were asked how family and friends respond to their work in corrections. The answers were mixed. Several of the women feel supported by those who are closest to them; others experience both positive and negative reactions; some receive no support in relation to this area of their lives. Some responses follow:

Some of my friends think that I'm daft because it's a dangerous situation. Some of my other friends are envious that I at least have an interesting job. My immediate family are split down the middle between thinking I'm daft and being envious. And my son thinks it's great!

My friends don't understand. My family accept it because I've been doing it for so long and I haven't been injured or taken hostage or anything. My husband has a totally dim view of corrections in general and he thinks I'm here for the money, I get no satisfaction out of it at all. In his words "it's something like being a whore, you do it for the money, you don't have to enjoy it." That's hard!!

Several of the women who participated in the project have had several years of experience in their jobs and appear largely to have overcome the barriers they faced. For some with less experience, as well as for some of the others, the jobs remain difficult and stressful.

In the next section, their stresses and coping mechanisms are discussed.

C   *Dealing with Stress*

This section explores women's responses to questions concerning how stressful they find the job, the causes of the stress and other related issues. Questions about the stress levels brought a range of responses. One woman responded as follows:

The job itself I don't find stressful. The staff I do. It seems to me the inmates the women can handle. They're not that demanding. The staff, I think, are more stressful. You are trying to dispel their questioning, their slurs as to whether or not you can do the job. That causes stress because you're constantly having to try to reaffirm that you are doing the job because they don't recognize that the job is being done and being done well. When I'm away from here I lift weights, I listen to music, do cross-country skiing, I try to keep busy.

The women were asked about the supports they have and who they talk to about the stress they are experiencing. Some responses follow:

I have a very good friend and we talk and talk and talk. I have a very close friend who is also in corrections and identifies with everything. We share things with each other that we share with no one else. If it weren't for her and I'm sure if it wasn't for me – for her – we would probably have a lot of problems.

The women were asked what would help them deal with the obstacles they face and what advice they would give to other women interested in working in corrections. Some of the respondants state that a supportive network of women in corrections would help them in dealing with the obstacles. A further suggestion is the need to educate male corrections workers about working with women. As for what they would say to other women, several mention the kind of qualities needed to work in the environment: maturity, strength, and self-assurance. These are necessary to withstand the difficulties they will face.

Examples of what is needed to overcome the obstacles that women face in this work include:

I think probably the men getting used to women being there a lot more. Women haven't been in our centre for that long and they still think of them as being separate. You get a couple of really good women in there, I think that would help them to see women as other staff rather than as women. Right now there's a lot of resentment on the part of the men that women are in there and they like to talk about the women.

Advice they would pass along includes:

She better be pretty strong. She'd better be very self-confident, very self-reliant and very mature. If you're not, then stay out because it will kill you, literally.

The women have had, and some continue to have, high levels of stress, not just because the job itself is stressful but because they are women leading the way in a very male-oriented atmosphere. They are resented by male corrections workers and are often greeted with hostility. Most of the women have dealt with some kind of harassment on the job. They have had to learn new coping skills, to become more assertive and to draw upon inner resources. There has been little assistance from within the system in helping them deal with a new environment.

The training women receive (if any) does not prepare them for the kind of hostility they will likely receive from their co-workers. Most of them receive support from their families and some get support from other women corrections workers and (occasionally) from male co-workers. It would seem that several who have worked in the system for a number of years meet with some measure of acceptance. As well, the women have made major adjustments in accommodating themselves to the correctional system. For some, as for the women in Sakowski's study, the costs have been high. In spite of the hardships described by the women who responded to the interview questions, it is apparent that many have learned to manage themselves very well and are making a real contribution to the correctional system. The maturity, strength, and competence they exhibit is impressive and admirable. Indeed, by their efforts, they have paved the way for other women to follow and for women to become integrated into an environment which they will help to shape in the future.

NOTES

1 The pilot study was funded by the President's Fund, University of Regina. The project was undertaken with Ron Schriml, School of Human Justice, University of Regina. Lynne Tony worked as research assistant.

REFERENCES

Armstrong, Pat and Hugh Armstrong 1984. *The Double Ghetto*. Toronto: McClelland and Stewart.

Baunach, Phyllis Jo 1982. "Sex-Role Operations." In Nicole Hahn Rafter and Elizabeth A. Stanko, eds., *Judge, Lawyer, Victim, Thief*. Boston: Northeastern University Press.

Bergen, Donna R. 1983. "Equality: Women in Corrections?" *Corrections Today* 45(5): 26–8, 36.

Bernard, Jessie 1971. *Women and the Public Interest*. Chicago/New York: Aldine-Atherton.

Braid, Kate 1976. "Women in Non-traditional Occupations in British Columbia." A preliminary study prepared for CSAA Annual General Meeting.

Bronskill, Ann 1980. "Female Correctional Officers in the Ministry of Correctional Services." On file, Ministry of Correctional Services, Government of Ontario, Toronto.

Chapman, Jane Roberts *et al.* 1980. *Women Employed in Corrections*. Center for Women Policy Studies.

Crouch, Ben M. 1985. "Pandora's Box: Women Guards in Men's Prisons." *Journal of Criminal Justice* 13: 535–48.

Eichler, Margrit 1980. *The Double Standard: A Feminist Critique of Feminist Social Science*. London: Croom Helm.

Feinman, Clarice 1980. *Women in the Criminal Justice System*. New York: Praeger Publishers.

Feinman, Clarice 1984. "Modesty or Muscle: Conflicting Views of the Role of Women Working in the Penal System." *Women in the Prison System*. Proceedings of Conference on Women in the Prison System, 12–14 June 1984, Australian Institute of Criminology.

Flynn, Edith Elizabeth 1982. "Women as Criminal Justice Professionals." In Nichole Hahn Rafter and Elizabeth A. Stanko, eds., *Judge, Lawyer, Victim, Thief*. Boston: Northeastern University Press.

Harm, Nancy J. 1981. "Female Employees in Male Institutions." In Barbara Hadley Olssen and Ann Dargis, eds., *Proceedings of the One Hundred and Tenth Annual Congress of Corrections*. College Park, Maryland: American Correctional Association.

Hartmann, Heidi 1979. "Capitalist Patriarchy and Job Segregation." In Zillah R. Eisenstein, ed., *Capitalist Patriarchy and the Case for Socialist Feminismn*. New York and London: Monthly Review Press.

Hillsman Baker, Sally 1978. "Women in Blue-Collar and Service Occupations." In Ann H. Stromberg and Shirley Harkness, eds., *Women Working: Theories and Facts in Perspective*. Palo Alto, California: Mayfield Publishing Co.

Jacobs, James B. 1979. "The Sexual Integration of the Prison's Guard Force: A Few Comments on Dothard V. Rawlinson." *University of Toledo Law Review* 10(2): 193–222.

Kissel, Peter and Paul L. Katsampes 1980. "The Impact of Women Corrections Officers on the Functioning of Institutions Housing Male Inmates." *Journal of Offender Counselling, Services and Rehabilitation* 4(3): 213–32.

Linden, Rich and Candice Minch 1982. *Women in Policing: A Review*. Winnipeg: The University of Manitoba.

Matthaei, Julie 1982. *An Economic History of Women in America*. New York: Schocken Books.

Matusewitch, Eric P. 1980. "Equal Opportunity for Female Correctional Officers: A Brief Overview." *Corrections Today* 42(6): 36–7.

Nicolia, Sandra 1981. "The Upward Mobility of Women in Corrections." In Robert Ross, ed., *Prison Guard/Correctional Officer – The Use and Abuse of Human Resources of Prisons*. Toronto: Butterworth.

O'Farrell, Bridgid and Shannon L. Harlan 1982. "Craftworkers and Clerks: The Effect of Male Co-workers Hostility on Women's Satisfaction with Non-traditional Jobs." *Social Problems* 29(3): 252–65.

Owen, Barbara 1985. "Race and Gender Relations Among Prison Workers." *Crime and Delinquency* 31(2): 147–259.

Phillips, Paul and Erin Phillips 1983. *Women and Work*. Toronto: James Lorimer.

Potter, Joan 1980 "Should Women Guards Work in Prisons for Men?" *Corrections Magazine* 6(5): 30–8.

Price, Barbara Raffel and Natalie J. Sokoloff 1982. *The Criminal Justice System and Women*. New York: Clark Boardman Co.

Rafter, Nicole Hahn and Elena M. Natalizia 1981. "Marxist Feminism: Implications for Criminal Justice." *Crime and Delinquency* 21(1): 81–98.

Riemer, Jeffrey W. and Lois Bridwell M. n.d. "How Women Survive in Non-traditional Occupations." Paper, Wichita State University, Department of Sociology.

Sakowski, Marie H. 1985–86. "Women Guards in Canada: A Study of the First Women to Work in a Federal Penitentiary for Male Offenders." *Resources for Feminist Research* 13(4): 52–3.

"Women in Combat Opposed." 1985. *The Leader Post*, Regina, Saskatchewan: Thursday, 23 May.

Women in Corrections 1981. American Correctional Association, College Park, Maryland, February.

Women, Minority Status, and Well-Being
Les femmes, leur situation minoritaire, et leur mieux-être

EVA A. SZEKELY

Immigrant Women and the Problem of Difference

Written from the standpoint of immigrant women, the main purpose of this paper is to demonstrate that "women's specificity" – women's work and values related to mothering and caring for others – is not an acceptable framework for analyzing the situations of immigrant women in Canada. Instead, one must begin by examining the complex interrelationships of employment, class structure, race/ethnicity, gender, and many other differences among women in an advanced capitalist country within a context of economic imperialism and neocolonialism. It is only when our differences are acknowledged and analyzed that adequate strategies for real equality can be formulated.[1]

Les immigrantes et le problème de la différence

Cet article rédigé du point de vue des immigrantes vise d'abord à démontrer que la « spécificité des femmes » – le travail et les valeurs des femmes par rapport au fait d'être mère et de prendre soin des autres – ne constitue pas un cadre valable pour l'analyse de la situation des immigrantes au Canada. Il faut plutôt commencer par examiner les interrelations complexes entre l'emploi, la structure des classes, « la race ou l'ethnie, » le sexe et de nombreuses autres différences chez les femmes vivant dans un pays capitaliste industrialisé, dans le contexte de l'impérialisme et du néocolonialisme. Ce n'est qu'une fois nos différences définies et analysées que nous pourrons élaborer des stratégies appropriées pour réaliser une égalité réelle.

I would like to address being different – being an immigrant woman – in a way that does not treat immigrant women as "objects of study"

or as an abstract category. I would like to write from what Dorothy
Smith (1987) described as the standpoint of women:

The standpoint of women ... can't be equated with perspective or worldview.
It does not universalize a particular experience. It is rather a method which,
at the outset of inquiry, creates a space for an absent subject and absent
experiences which is to be filled with the presence and spoken experience
of actual women speaking of and in the actualities of their everyday worlds.
(Smith 1987, 3)

I want to create such a space for absent subjects and absent experiences. The inquiry must begin with the experiences of real,
embodied subjects, and it must explain how our experiences are
"knitted into the extended social relations of a contemporary capitalist economy and society" (Smith 1987, 5). When we speak of immigrant women, we must consider their experiences in the light of
at least *two* sets of extended social relations – not only the current
social relations in Canada but also those in the women's countries
of origin. The experiences of immigrant women are historical, dynamic, and ever changing, as are the social relations from which
their daily lives are inseparable.

How do we make this space? How do we preserve the presence
of actual subjects? I am one of those subjects whose presence I want
to preserve. I want to include my experiences without universalizing
them, without implying that this is what all immigrant women experience in Canada. As a white, educated person I am a privileged
immigrant. Despite my privileged position, however, I have felt that
I am – I am treated as – different.

In *The Voyage of the Damned*, a movie chronicling the events of 1939
that forced the steamship *St. Louis* to return to Europe with its 937
passengers, two-thirds of whom eventually died in concentration
camps, the German steward asked one of the passengers: "What
does it feel like to be a Jew in Germany?" The former concentration
camp inmate answered, "It is to be reminded of it every day." Although I have not experienced what it was like to be a Jew in Nazi
Germany, these words described perfectly a set of experiences I do
know: the experiences of being immigrant.

"It is to be reminded of it" – of being different, of being immigrant
– every day. I want to use the word "immigrant" not to describe a
person, but to designate a position that has been created by social
practices and policies. Instead of asking "what is an immigrant" I
want to ask, as Jean-Paul Sartre asked concerning Jews, how is an
immigrant *made*? About Jews he had this to say:

It is neither their past, their religion, nor their soil that unites the sons [sic] of Israel. If they have a common bond, if all of them deserve the name of Jew, it is because they have in common the *situation* of a Jew, that is, they live in a community which *takes them for Jews*. (Sartre 1946/1974, 67; my emphases).

The term "immigrant" is applied to individuals each of whom has a different identity and social history. My discussion primarily concerns women emigrating from Third World countries and southern Europe and secondarily concerns Canadian-born visible minorities. Not all people who are technically or legally immigrant are identified or identify themselves as such. Most immigrants from the United States and Great Britain are two obvious examples. Similarly, one may be Canadian-born and -raised and still be treated as an immigrant. Japanese and Chinese Canadians and other visible minorities, for example, are often seen as immigrants (Das Gupta 1986; Ng and Estable 1987). These persons only become immigrant as a result of definite social processes that stamp them with the identification immigrant, which is synonymous with "ethnically and racially inferior" (Bodnar 1983, 8).

Unfortunately, this process is nothing new. In December 1943, people could read the following in the *Toronto Star*:

The Canadian Legion has always taken the stand [that] the admission of immigrants to Canada should be carefully regulated with a view to giving preference to people of British stock or of other nations who share our democratic ideals and can be readily assimilated into our national life. (*Toronto Star*, 2 Aug. 1987, B1).

We can find reports of racism in Canada from centuries ago. Documents from 1628 suggest that early in the seventeenth century, Quebec tried to solve the problems of its inadequate labour force by slavery (Head 1981). The Chinese Exclusion Act, which was in effect from 1923 until 1947, barred entry to all Chinese people with the exception of students and merchants. In 1939 Canada was one of the countries that refused entry to the 937 Jews on board the *St. Louis*, while British women and children were welcomed excitedly as "our little war guests" (*Toronto Star*, 2 August 1987).

Even these few examples from Canada's racist immigration history illustrate that, like a Jew, an immigrant is *made*. Like the Jew, the immigrants I am discussing are often treated as foreign intruders, representatives of alien races, strange religions, threatening political views. It is for these reasons that the immigrant is, like the Jew,

considered virtually unassimilable (cf., Sartre 1974, 100). If she or
he is not to act in bad faith, (Sartre 1972) an immigrant cannot
choose not to be an immigrant, the same way as a Jew cannot choose
not to be a Jew (Sartre 1974, 136).

When I seek to accept my immigrant position, I must acknowledge
a number of *other* positions with which it is intertwined. At a job
interview I had a few years ago these other positions were brought
under scrutiny as well. I was grilled for *what kind* of an immigrant
I was – politically on the right or on the left? I was grilled on my
religious views. In the sixth hour of the interview I confessed to
being on the left and being an atheist of Jewish Hungarian parents.
I did not have to confess to being a woman; I was treated as one
from the moment I arrived. My skin colour and academic qualifications were obvious; those constituted my privileged status. In this
situation, all I had against me were my political and (lack of) religious
views, my being a woman of Jewish parents, and my speaking with
an accent.

I choose this example to illustrate that when someone fills the
position of immigrant, she simultaneously stands in many other positions as well. I would like to emphasize that in the example I
provided, as I believe in most other cases, being a woman was only
one of them. Scrutiny of the potential and already admitted immigrant's skin colour or national origin and political and religious views
is inseparable from Canada's trying to maintain a social-political-
economic order built on a system of exploitation. This function of
immigration policies and practices, however, remains concealed
from many Canadian people.

One effect of this concealment is that immigrants are blamed for
the country's growing unemployment rates, for poverty among
Canadian-born people, and for what is seen as excessive welfare
budgets spent largely on immigrants and their children (*Toronto Star*,
26 April 1987). As Irving Abella put it, "we are a nation full of
immigrants that hates immigrants." To many Canadians, he added,
"this country is starting to look like the United Nations, and they
are not sure they like seeing faces of other colors next to them on
the street or the subway" (*Toronto Star*, 2 August 1987).

Another effect is that many Canadians find it difficult to understand why it is that some immigrants continue to discuss and try to
influence the social and political life of what continues to feel like
the home country. Perhaps it is even more disconcerting to many
Canadians that immigrants criticize social and political life in Canada
from a foreign perspective, and some immigrants want to see the
kinds of changes in Canada that they hoped to accomplish back

home. Although our experiences of immigration have undoubtedly
changed us, they did not make us anew. These experiences did not
erase our previous ways of thinking, feeling, and acting. We carry
within us, and in some ways we continue to be, everything that we
were before coming to Canada (cf. Disman 1976).

It does a disservice to those of us who are immigrants to deny that
we are different. We *are* different as a group, insofar as our social
and personal histories were formed outside Canada. We cannot
share Canada's past; we did not participate in the experiences of
this country's people. Because of this, wrote Alfred Schuetz (1944/
1960, 103), the immigrant is a person "without a history." But there
is another sense in which the immigrant is someone without a history.
In most cases, we cannot share our own past either. It is nearly
impossible to share our histories when Canadian history texts rarely
give more than superficial mention to immigrants, when we are
absent or portrayed as people without roots. As Bannerji (1987, 10)
points out, even the "Women's Studies curriculum leaves the reader
with the impression that women from the Third World and Southern
Europe are a very negligible part of the living and labouring population in Canada." This is another reason why it is so difficult for
persons in the position immigrant to become part of Canadian society. Being without a history in these two senses is the basis of the
profound sense of isolation and loneliness that many of us experience (Szekely 1987).

As individuals we are also very different from one another. What
we do have in common is being immigrants and women, but because
of our racial or ethnic, political, religous, and other differences our
situations differ greatly. We cannot simply say that all immigrant
women have a common lot – or a common enemy. In terms of
employment, for example, immigrant women constitute two distinct
groups in Canada. One group of immigrant women work in well
paid professional or managerial jobs, while women in the other much
larger group are among the lowest paid and most exploited workers.
These differences in occupation, educational level, and income have
been documented by several authors (Boyd 1986; Estable 1986;
Arnopoulos 1979).

WOMEN'S SPECIFICITY?

How, then, can we analyze the situations of immigrant women in
Canada? The method of analysis is crucial because of its implications
for what can and should be done to improve their lives. One possible
method of analysis would be to start with the notion of women's

specificity. In Angela Miles's (1982) discussion of this notion, women's specificity refers to women's specific experiences of, and responsibilities for, reproduction; it refers to women's work and values related to the experiences of mothering and caring for others.

If we were to start from this analytic framework, we would have to add on other descriptors immediately to accommodate the *specifities* of women *within* the position immigrant. If we begin with women's specificity, all other differences among women would be rendered secondary, that is, less important. Yet it can be argued that the racial or ethnic, political, economic, educational, geographic, age, and language-related differences are no less important than our specific experiences as women. To base the analysis on women's responsibility for, and experiences of, reproduction is to run the risk of reducing women to their biological functions. Most importantly, however, to designate as the primary analytic category women's work and values related to reproduction is not to see gender as only *one* of many intertwining dimensions of people's lives.

However tempting it may be, our differences as immigrant women cannot be explained and should not be treated as cultural. R. Ng (1979, 1981) and Reimer (1980) have demonstrated that it is by using particular interpretive procedures that what are actually class relations come to be located in family traditions, which are then attributed to the cultural backgrounds of the immigrant families (Reimer 1980, 31). This state of affairs is not unique to Canada. Researchers in European countries have observed that in Western Europe migrant women "live and work under conditions closest to the working class. But the constraints on the choices open to them are so great that they often appear marginal to it" (Morokvasic 1981). Due to legal, linguistic, and racist barriers, it is difficult for immigrant women (and men) in Europe and Canada to recognize the interests they have in common with working-class women and men and to organize around these interests.

Similarly, class relations are not part of the ways in which many Canadians, including helping professionals, view the problems immigrant women face. The problems are conceptualized as ethnic in origin, which implies solutions of a similar character. Neither during nor after their training are most professionals encouraged to discuss and seek to understand how emotional and physical illnesses are created by specific economic and social conditions. In the absence of such training it is not surprising that the proposed solutions for the illnesses women suffer are "personal or cultural, focused on helping a women 'cope' with a bad situation, rather than focusing outward to find ways to change this situation" (Bodnar 1983, 10).

In the case of immigrant women, then, the solution may be to observe traditions within the family (often what the mental health professional may think the traditions are) and to try to adapt and integrate into the Canadian way of life outside the family – a rather schizoid solution.

It is only when class differences are construed as cultural or ethnic differences that the call of agencies and institutions to help immigrants adapt makes any sense (cf. Head 1981; Ontario Economic Council 1970). It is only when the analytic concepts of class and exploitation are concealed and replaced by concepts such as "value differences" or "culture clash" that immigrant can be blamed for failing to assimilate into Canadian society.[2]

How does it happen that class remains hidden and instead culture appears as the essence of difference between immigrants and the Canadian-born? Class and class structure remain hidden, at least in part, by concealing the fact that immigrant women *work for wages*. Immigrant women as workers are largely invisible. We rarely read or hear about them in the popular media. Yet the majority of immigrant women are not housewives. The immigration agencies treat them as such, by not assessing their skills when they enter the country as sponsored immigrants and by not providing adequate opportunities for training in language and job skills (WWIW Brief 1986).

Despite their obvious disadvantages, however, a larger proportion of immigrant women are employed than Canadian-born women.[3] This statement does *not*, however, corroborate the main finding of a recent study by Seward and McDade (1988, 8) namely that, in almost every respect, immigrant women, as a group, appear to be doing better economically than Canadian-born women." Census data indicate that most of them work in the lowest paying, dead-end jobs. While on the average the statistics *may* support this 1988 report's general statement, figures based on aggregates of post-war immigration present a distorted view of most immigrant women's actual life situations today. Recent (1976–81) immigrant women's average incomes were, in fact, $1,500 lower than for the previous group (1971–75) of immigrant women (see p. 12 of the report). Yet no questions were asked about how the higher averages came about; there is nothing in the report to indicate that many immigrant women are working in several part-time, low-paying jobs with no security or benefits.

When we examine Canada's immigration policies and practices it becomes evident that the concealment of class differences (the maintenance of a certain political-economic order) is inseparable from the racism characteristic of our society. The pivot of this connection

is work or employment.[4] Since the late 1960s, under the family class
or sponsored category, increasing numbers of unskilled women have
also been admitted to fill the demand for low-wage jobs. Since the
late 1970s the number of domestic workers has increased substantially as well.[5] Many of these women are from the Caribbean and
the Philippines; half of them work as live-in domestics, with little or
no protection under labour standards legislation (Ramirez 1984).
Domestic workers can obtain landed immigrant status only with great
difficulty. Because of their working conditions, most domestic workers cannot fulfill Immigration's requirement of "self-sufficiency" to
achieve landed status and to bring their families to the country.

    Though they are not immigrants in the legal sense, the situation
of foreign domestic workers must be included in any discussion of
immigrant women, for two reasons. First, domestic workers need
support to obtain legal and labour rights. Secondly, their situation
shows most clearly that immigration policies are directed toward
filling "Canadian labour market shortages" (Toronto *Globe and Mail*,
19 September 1988, A4) by obtaining cheap labour. It is a way to
keep some people down – or out – and to ensure the relatively free
movement of capital. As Himani Bannerji (1987, 10) noted, it is a
way to continue to create "a working class ... through racist immigration policies and segmentation of the labour market ... where a
U.S. dependent capitalism has long entered an imperialist phase."
Racist practices, as we well know, are not limited to immigration
policies and processes. Quite likely, white members of our society
may not have dealt with their "common sense racism," as Bannerji
(1987) pointed out, adding that

It is perhaps for this reason that the racism of the left feminists is almost
always of omission rather than that of commission. They probably truly
cannot *see* us or why it is that racism and "ethnicity" are integral to the study
of women in Canada – even when they study the area of labour/capital
relations, i.e., class. And those feminists who do see us or that racism is an
issue very often deal with it in the spirit of Christian humanism, on the
ground of morality and doing good, or in the spirit of bourgeois democracy,
which "includes" or adds on representatives from the "minority" communities (Bannerji 1987, 11).

Immigrant women who work with Third World and Southern European women are aware of many white feminists' inability to really
see "immigrant" women in their actual life situations. These women
are deeply aware of the class differences between themselves and
white middle-class feminists. As one of them stated, "white women

do the talking, while immigrant women roll up their sleeves and work." Several immigrant women have pointed out that white feminists often fail to understand how immigrant women operate. Many immigrant women are intimidated by the differences in talk and by the ways in which white feminists run their meetings (W. Ng 1982, 253). They point out that white feminists are all too willing to "take on leadership roles and to give directions to immigrant women about how to organize."

Immigrant women feel that there is a division in terms of language as well. White feminists, as one woman said, "speak differently, they are more articulate" and, she added, "they are so wrapped up in analyzing that they often can't hear what immigrant women have to say." They can't hear, for example, that many immigrant women are truly afraid to speak, afraid that they might be deported, remarked one women. They can't hear, said a woman who has been in Canada for nearly twenty years, that "immigrant women still face the same problems as ten years ago." White feminists, she added, "still don't see how immigration agencies, work places, and health care systems treat immigrant women." Immigrant women continue to struggle virtually without support against sponsorship and the problems related to it. The same woman also noted that feminist groups have often forgotten to advertise marches and demonstrations for causes that are also of concern to immigrant women in languages other than English. Finally, many immigrants resent the patronizing attitude they perceive, even among progressive people; they resent being mentally colonized, and being made to feel grateful for having been admitted to Canada, noted one woman.

These comments by immigrant women in Canada are consistent with Bannerji's description of common sense racism and with its corollary, the insufficient support for racial and ethnic minorities. Bannerji, of course, rejects any analysis of gender that severs the interrelationships of gender with class and race. Such analyses, she writes,

empty out gender relations of their general social context, content and dynamism. This, along with the primacy that gender gains (since the primary social determinant is perceived as patriarchy) subsumes all other social relations, indeed renders them often invisible. The particular – i.e., one moment – begins to stand for the whole (Bannerji 1987, 12).

I believe that Bannerji's position is correct. If indeed patriarchy were the primary determinant guiding social relations, how would we explain the oppression and exploitation of women by women? How, then, could the foreign domestics' work and life situations persist in the households of many Canadian women? A framework that purports to explain a woman's subordination must be able to handle these events in the lives of women, whether they work as domestics, whether they are Canadian-born or immigrant working-class women, or whether they are the indigenous women of Canada.

WHAT IS TO BE DONE?

The main purpose of my paper has been to demonstrate that the situations of immigrant women in Canada must be understood in the complex interrelationships of employment, class structure, race and ethnicity, and gender, as well as of other differences among women. The interrelationships of these differences have to be examined within a state capitalist economy that has been heavily – and, with the threat of Free Trade, increasingly – dependent on the United States. This is no small task, but we have no alternatives if our aim is to transform the situations in which women have been oppressed and exploited. The women's movement in Canada is just beginning to take up "the causes of women who are not white and not middle class" (Bodnar 1983, 8), and we have a long way to go yet. Immigrant women's organizations clearly want and need the support of white feminist groups. The issue for feminist groups is what kind of support can and should they offer, and how should it be done.

We must begin with the recognition, as Mariana Valverde (1982, 301) noted, that

women are oppressed in different ways, apart from all being oppressed as women. Immigrant women have to be organized as immigrant women, and *then* plug into the women's movement. It would be very alienating for individual immigrant women to join a group that was primarily anglo. They need their own groups, which fight for specifically immigrant women's issues and identify their own concerns, so that when they come into the general women's movement they can set their own demands.

One issue that immediately arises is funding; immigrant women's groups have been chronically underfunded. Feminist groups could lobby for the establishment of more government programs to provide core funding for immigrant women's groups (cf. wwiw Brief 1986).

Immigrant women's groups initiate programs of their own because the governments do not meet even their most basic needs. Translation and interpretation services are practically nonexistent (*Toronto*

Star, 18 September 1988, A1, A6). Training in the English language and in job skills with living allowance and child care; supporting immigrant women's organizations in their struggles against sponsorship, which creates "second class citizens" (wwiw Brief 1986); struggles for higher minimum wages, for health care and counselling services, for language training in the work place, for better occupational safety standards and their enforcement, are further examples. Feminists in academic circles could analyze the implications for immigrant women, of the particular research and theoretical work that is being conducted within their fields of study. They could identify the kinds of research and the methods that would foster the transformation of immigrant women's situations. They could support immigrant women's groups to do their *own* research and policy analyses about matters of their lives (Szekely 1988).

Even this brief list of potential areas of action by feminist groups in support of immigrant women leaves us with infinite tasks. All of these tasks are interrelated; to work on any one of them is to give a push – however small – to all the others. If we are willing to learn from immigrant and other minority women about their situations and if we learn to work together, some day all women might truly be different – but equal.

NOTES

1 I would like to thank the immigrant women who have generously shared their experiences for the purposes of writing this paper. Special thanks are due to Salome Loucas for helpful suggestions and numerous discussions on immigrant women. Acknowledgements are also due to the Canadian Research Institute for the Advancement of Women for financial assistance.

2 The importance of issues of class and the class structure of Canadian society in understanding the problems immigrant women face underlies Roxana Ng and Alma Estable's (1987) paper, "Immigrant Women in the Labour Force" and of Monica Boyd's (1986) chapter, "Immigrant Women in Canada."

3 Immigrant women's participation in the paid labour force has been, and continues to be, higher than that of Canadian-born women – 55.6 per cent as compared to 52.1 per cent (Estable 1986). This statistic does not include the unknown numbers of immigrant women who work on an occasional or regular basis for cash.

4 In the 1950s and 1960s large numbers of highly educated male and female immigrants were accepted into Canada due to the country's need for more professionals and scientists. (We should note that Canada's growing

need for professionals and scientists coincided with a "brain-drain" from Canada to the United States – that is, the country's employment and immigration needs have not been independent of Canada's ties with the United States.) During this period, one-third of all immigrants were from the United Kingdom and only one of ten immigrants were born outside Europe (Estable 1986).

5 In 1983 alone 35,000 women were issued temporary work permits (Estable 1986) to do the jobs that most Canadian women and men will not take. Unknown numbers of women work as illegal domestics, without work permits. These undocumented women are particularly exploited by their employers, since they have no protection at all in Canada (Cohen 1987). Women in neither group show up in immigration statistics since most of them are here only temporarily.

REFERENCES

Arnopoulos, S. McLeod 1979. "Problems of Immigrant Women in the Canadian Labour Force." Ottawa: Canadian Advisory Council on the Status of Women.

Bannerji, H. 1987. "Introducing Racism: Notes towards an Anti-racist Feminism," *Resources for Feminist Research* 1: 10–12.

Bodnar, A. 1986. "Realities for Immigrant Women: O Canada! Not Home and Native Land," *Broadside* 4: 8–10.

Boyd, M. 1986. "Immigrant Women in Canada." In R.J. Simon and C.B. Brettell, eds., *International Migration: The Female Experience.* Ottawa, N.J.: Rowman and Allanheld.

Cohen, R. 1987. "The Work Conditions of Immigrant Women Live-in Domestics: Racism, Sexual Abuse and Invisibility." *Resources for Feminist Research* 1: 36–38.

Das Gupta, T. 1986. *Learning From Our History: Community Development by Immigrant Women in Ontario 1958–1986.* Toronto: Cross Cultural Communication Centre.

Disman, M. 1976. "Omnia Mea Mecum Porto (Everything That I Have I am Carrying with Me): My Experience of Immigration." *Reflections* 2: 57–80.

Estable, A. 1986. "Immigrant Women in Canada – Current Issues." Ottawa: Canadian Advisory Council on the Status of Women.

Head, W. 1981. "Adaptation of Immigrants in Metro Toronto: Perceptions of Ethnic and Racial Discrimination." Toronto: York University.

Miles, A. 1982. "Ideological Hegemony in Political Discourse: Women's Specificity and Equality." In A. Miles and G. Finn, eds., *Feminism in Canada.* Montreal: Black Rose Books.

Morokvasic, M. 1981. "The Invisible Ones: A Double Role of Women in the Current European Migrations." In L. Eitinger and D. Schwartz, eds., *Strangers in the World*. Bern: Hans Huber Publishers.

Ng, R. 1979. "Services to Immigrant Women: A Critical Analysis." Paper presented at the Canadian Sociology and Anthropology Association Annual Meeting, Saskatoon.

Ng, R. 1981. "Constituting Ethnic Phenomenon: An Account from the Perspective of Immigrant Women." *Canadian Ethnic Studies* 1: 97–108.

Ng, R. and A. Estable 1987. "Immigrant Women in the Labour Force: An Overview of Present Knowledge and Research Gaps." *Resources for Feminist Research* 1: 29–33.

Ng, Winnie. 1982. "Immigrant Women: The Silent Partners." In M. FitzGerald, M. Wolfe and C. Guberman, eds., *Still Ain't Satisfied!*. Toronto: Women's Press.

Ontario Economic Council 1970. "Immigrant Integration." (Report).

Ramirez, J. 1984. "Good Enough to Stay." *Currents* 1.

Reimer, M. 1980. "Constituting Class as Cultural Difference." Paper presented at the Learned Society, Sociology Section, Session on Women and Ethnicity, Montreal.

Sartre, J.-P. 1946/1974. *Anti-semite and Jew*. New York: Schocken.

Sartre, J.-P. 1972. *Being and Nothingness*. New York: Washington Square Press.

Schuetz, A. 1944/1960. "The Stranger: An Essay in Social Psychology." In M.R. Stein, A.J. Vidich, and D.M. White, eds., *Identity and Anxiety*. New York: The Free Press.

Seward, S. and K. McDade 1988. "Immigrant Women in Canada: A Policy Perspective." Ottawa: Canadian Advisory Council on the Status of Women.

Smith, D.E. 1987. *The Everyday World as Problematic: A Sociology from the Standpoint of Women*. Toronto: University of Toronto Press.

Szekely, E. 1987. "The Stranger: A Critical Exposition of Alfred Schuetz's Essay in Social Psychology." Paper presented at the Annual Meeting of the Ontario Psychological Association, Toronto.

Szekely, E. 1988. "Immigrant Women in Canada: A Policy Perspective – New Study by CACSW." *Women Working with Immigrant Women Newsletter*, Spring.

Valverde, M. 1982. "What Are Our Options?" In M. FitzGerald, M. Wolfe, and C. Guberman, eds., *Still Ain't Satisfied!* Toronto: Women's Press.

Women Working With Immigrant Women 1986. "Sponsorship Concerns, Funding Concerns, Health, Education, and Labour Needs of Immigrant Women." Brief presented to the Policy Directors of the Ministries of Health, Labour, Education, Skills Development, Citizenship and Culture, Industry, Trade and Technology, Treasury and Economy, Toronto.

KABAHENDA NYAKABWA AND CAROL D.H. HARVEY

Adaptation to Canada: The Case of Black Immigrant Women

Adaptation is the process of establishing a relatively stable and reciprocal relationship with the environment in which immigrants find themselves. All immigrants experience serious hardships as they enter the job market due to language problems, non-recognition of qualifications, lack of necessary licences, lack of Canadian experience, and direct discrimination. Immigrant women are doubly disadvantaged because of their sex and countries of origin. But the double disadvantage becomes a triple jeopardy for black immigrant women, since they must also face the pervasive racism of Canadian society. Their social networks are deficient, their life satisfaction is low, and they suffer from emotional isolation.

L'adaptation au Canada: le cas des immigrantes noires

L'adaptation est le processus par lequel une immigrante établit des relations stables et réciproques avec l'environnement dans lequel elle se trouve. Les immigrantes vivent des expériences pénibles sur le marché du travail à cause de difficultés occasionnées par la langue, le fait que leurs diplômes ne soient pas reconnus, l'absence de permis d'exercer leur profession, le manque d'expérience canadien ne pertinente et la discrimination directe. Les femmes immigrantes sont défavorisées à cause de leur sexe et de leur pays d'origine, mais quand il s'agit des immigrantes noires, le double handicap devient triple car en plus elles doivent affronter le racisme de la société canadienne. Leurs réseaux sociaux sont insuffisants, elle ne sont pas satisfaites de leur vie et elles souffrent d'isolement émotif.

When people migrate to a new country, resettlement involves a process of adaptation. Not only does the newcomer have to take action which can objectively be recognized as adapting to the new culture, such as getting a job and finding housing, but the person also thinks of the new surroundings and reacts to them subjectively. In this paper we will consider the issues and problems that arise for a special case of newcomers, black African women. We will demonstrate how their experiences are similar to, as well as different from, those of other newcomers to Canada. We will also suggest ways to facilitate their adaptation, through research, social policy, and collective actions of the women themselves.

REVIEW OF THE LITERATURE

To study the special case of black African immigrants, we need to put their experiences in the context of social science research. Accordingly, we have reviewed the literature on immigrants and refugees as it applies to black African women. It is also important to put the research in a theoretical framework, and we have chosen family stress theory as suitable for this purpose.

Definition of Terms

Newcomers may come to Canada as voluntary migrants, mainly for work, and are classified as immigrants by the government. Technically, immigrants enter Canada with citizenship from another country. If they qualify as immigrants, they may be classified as permanent residents and participate fully in the economic and social life of the country.

Black African women can immigrate under different legal categories. One of the most common is that of assisted relative, which means that a woman was allowed to enter because she had a relative in Canada willing to sponsor her. Included are "siblings, parents, grandparents less than 60 years of age, married daughters, nieces, aunts, or grandchildren of the sponsor" (Manitoba Employment Services and Economic Security 1983, 52). Another common entry is as part of a family class, which includes "sponsored spouses, fiancées, unmarried children under 21, and grandparents over 60" (Manitoba Employment Services and Economic Security 1983, 53). Many immigrant non-white women "come to Canada with their husbands to fill the most menial, unskilled sectors of the labour market, doing work that other Canadians do not want to do" (Bannerji et al. 1987, 3).

An African woman may also come to Canada as a refugee, sponsored by the government, a private group, or an individual. In this case too she may come alone or as part of a family group. In contrast to assisted relatives, refugees have fled homelands, often in haste and in fear of their lives. They often have had to leave family members behind to uncertain fates; in additional, refugees may not have had much choice in selecting the country of resettlement (Copeland and Harvey 1986).

Immigrants may also come to Canada if they have a job waiting for them or have sufficient income to employ people in a private business. These people migrate to improve their economic positions, and they are free to go back to their countries of origin, while refugees often cannot (Copeland and Harvey 1986). Few black African women come to Canada under this last category.

Regardless of the category of entry, immigrants and refugees have to make changes to be able to function in the country of resettlement. Called adaptation by social scientists and lay people alike, the changes occur over time and are part of a process. Adaptation processes involve establishing a relatively stable and reciprocal relationship with their surroundings and having meaningful human, social, and interpersonal relationships with the community (Brody 1970).

Adaptation is both objective and subjective. Objective adaptation involves participating in the economic and social system as shown by getting a job or belonging to a formal organization. Subjective adaptation is an internal process whereby the newcomer begins to identify with the new country and to be committed to it, indicated by feelings of being at home and having family and neighbouring relationships (Richmond 1974).

Family Stress Theory

In order to put the many factors associated with adaptation of immigrants and refugees into perspective, it is useful to examine family stress theory. Family stess may be defined as "an upset in the steady state of the family" (Boss 1987). Migration, by definition, causes an upset to families and individuals. They encounter a new physical environment as well as a new social system, which may or may not be similar to the one they have left.

In studying war-separated American families, Hill (1949) proposed an ABCX model of family stress. He said that three classes of variables were important to predict the level of stress on the family: the stressor event (A); the resources (B) the family possesses or develops to deal with the stressor; and (C), the perception that individuals or families develop about the meaning of the stressor event. These three variables interact to produce a given level of stress or crisis, (X). This model has been used by social scientists studying family reactions to stress and has been modified to include changes in the family over time (McCubbin and Patterson in 1983 proposed a double-ABCX model). It is appropriate to classify variables in migration research found to affect black African women as they come to Canada.

The advantage of using this stress model is that we can account for both objective adaptation (resources, B in the model) and subjective adaptation (definition, C in the model). Further, we can observe different types of migration and classification of immigration status (the stressor event and factors surrounding it, A in the model), and we can specify how these interact to produce a given level of stress or adaptation to Canada (X in the model). We can consider the adaptation process over time by applying McCubbin and Patterson's 1983 refinement to Hill's model. We can thus predict that adaptation can be "bon" or "mal," using McCubbin and Patterson's (1983) terms, and that it can change over time as new resources are developed or new perceptions of the country of resettlement are formed.

This paper is therefore organized into parts that group the variables found by researchers to influence adaptation by immigrants into three classes: the original event (moving) and the factors which surround it, such as immigration status; resources which the person may possess or acquire in order to adapt; and subjective interpretation of the new country. All of these factors are influenced by attitudes and laws of the new country, which we will also consider from a Canadian context. Taken together, these variables will interact to produce bon or maladaptation of the newcomer, following the double-ABCX theory.

MOVING AND IMMIGRATION STATUS

Voluntary migrant, sponsored family member, or refugee – each classification has different consequences for the newcomer. Those who come as voluntary migrants do not have to worry about family members' safety at home, and they know that if they have enough money they can contact or visit their homeland. Sponsored family members have relatives already established in Canada and thus may have a home ready for them. Refugees have to make abrupt changes and may not have had a chance to consider carefully Canada as a place to resettle. Thus the classifications under which a woman enters Canada will affect her chances for work or study.

In addition, immigration status has an effect on retirement benefits. Women who are admitted to Canada under the family class or assisted relative category do not have the same rights as other immigrants. They do not have access to student loans and bursaries, and they are not eligible to claim allowances for language or skill training. They do not have access to welfare benefits for a period of at least five years, or, in the case of family class, as long as ten years, depending on the financial situation of the guarantor (Personal interview with Manitoba immigration officer, 27 July 1987).

RESOURCE POSSESSION AND DEVELOPMENT

The newcomer will come with resources, both financial and social, and may also develop new resources over time in the new country. Of the many resources that have been investigated by social scientists, we chose to concentrate on those which have been found to be most influential during successful adaptation: employment, language fluency, family interaction, and health.

Employment

Studies of immigrants show that successful employment is a key variable. Most immigrants experience serious employment hardships (Boyd 1984; Montero 1979; Neuwirth 1987; Richmond 1984; Samuel 1984). Obstacles to achieving satisfactory employment include language problems, lack of necessary licences, unwillingness of the government to recognize qualifications, lack of work experience in Canada, and/or direct discrimination (Richmond 1984, 20), particularly against visible minorities (Burke 1984).

Immigrant women tend to work in both the highest and the lowest ranges of the labour market, with little representation in between (Estable 1986, 20). They are under-represented in white collar jobs and over-represented in blue collar occupations (Boyd 1984). A dismal picture of the employment of immigrant women is painted in the literature, researchers find that these workers are poorly paid, working as domestics, chambermaids, waitresses, and sewing machine operators. As such, they are often "ignored by unions and inadequately protected by provincial legislation" (Arnopolous 1979, 3).

The reasons for such low-status employment for the average woman immigrant are several. First, the job market is sex-segregated, and thus jobs are more readily available in clerical and service positions as well as in particular industrial categories such as textiles (Bodner and Reimer 1981). Second, women vary in their educational levels and occupational skills (Estable 1986, 21). Third, language barriers prevent employment in many jobs and channel many immigrant women into job ghettoes such as the garment industry, where "they are subject to hazardous and exploitative working conditions, long hours, and very poor wages, especially those doing piece-work at home" (Estable 1986, 26). Fourth, Canada or the province may not recognize licences or other qualifications obtained in the country of origin. Often these women accept employment below their level of qualification (Estable 1986), experiencing occupational deflection.

Immigrant women also suffer from higher rates of unemployment than Canadian-born women (Estable 1986). This is in part due to employment in low status occupations, which have more frequent layoffs. It is also due to difficulties in presenting their skills to prospective employers and in negotiating wages and work schedules (Ng 1984, 216). Furthermore, lack of skill in English or French may mean employment in low status, frequently laid-off positions (Estable 1986).

Language Fluency

Lack of knowledge of one of the official languages of Canada creates difficulties in employment and in other areas of social life. An immigrant woman who cannot speak English or French cannot communicate in her neighbourhood, making it hard for her to shop, go to the hospital, or visit with others. In the long run, she may even become alienated from family members as her husband at work or children at school gain fluency. The woman may thus become dependent on family members to interpret the culture to her, and children may even become gatekeepers of information, changing family role positions (Chan and Lam 1983; Huyck and Fields 1981; Taft and Johnson 1967).

Immigrant women could benefit from language classes, but these are often offered in the evenings. After a day of hard work on the job, tired from household chores, many immigrant women, especially those with small children, find it hard to attend language classes. Moreover, language training available is often part-time, inappropriate, or rudimentary (Estable 1986, 45).

It is important to remember that age of migration is important to the acquisition of a new language. For example, Montero (1979, 111) reports that an old woman said, "I went to English class but it was very difficult. My tongue and my head are not built for strange new sounds".

Family Interaction

Like other Canadians, immigrant women are assigned roles at work and at home, making long hours necessary. In addition, family values and attitudes of the home country may conflict with those of Canada.

If married to a man who expects a clear sex-linked division of labour together with male authority, she may experience conflicts as she begins to accept Canadian values. If she begins to think that women's status is equal to men's or if she wants both husband and wife to share in domestic responsibilities, he may think she is showing disrespect for him. To question traditional values may create tension in families and lead to divorce, alcoholism, or wife abuse. Role changes brought about by children acting as gatekeepers, as mentioned above, may also create family tensions.

For women who come to Canada alone, finding mates can be difficult as well, particularly for visible minorities. If one is lucky enough to be part of a large ethnic community, this may not be such a problem. For Africans, who are few in number anyway and who come from many countries and ethnic groups, finding an appropriate mate is more difficult. Women may feel constrained to pick a partner who is acceptable by standards applicable at home by (for example) marrying within the proper clan or tribe; to violate those expectations by marrying an outsider is to incur criticism from families at home.

Health

Both physical and mental health may be problematic for the immigrant woman. As mentioned above, language barriers may make it difficult to discuss complaints with medical personnel. Furthermore, these women must know how to gain access to the medical system. Women may be reluctant to discuss certain aspects of their anatomy with male medical personnel, and they may not want their children to interpret for them.

Mental health may also be difficult to maintain. Physicians may consider mental health problems to be merely a lack of adjustment, and they may not treat the immigrant woman properly (Bodner and Reimer 1981, 51). Her problems may be seen as individual rather than as a result of environmental pressure. Individualized solutions may then be applied, such as prescribing a tranquilizing drug, rather than helping her with language or employment difficulties.

SUBJECTIVE INTERPRETATIONS

Not only do the conditions of her immigration and the possession of resources affect the adjustment of an immigrant, but subjective interpretations are also important. Evaluation of one's quality of life is complex, resulting from the interplay between objective conditions and subjective feelings about them (Rogers and Converse 1975). Quality of life includes satisfaction of one's basic physical, biological, psychological, economic and social needs (Bubolz, Eicher, Evers and Sontag 1980).

Satisfaction with the new culture thus depends somewhat on objective conditions, such as having a job, but it also depends on having friends or work colleagues to help interpret the new culture. People who can make friends, who interact with the ethnic community from the country of origin, and who can communicate with members of the dominant culture are in a position to gain help with their subjective interpretations (Copeland and Harvey 1989).

FACTORS IN THE NEW COUNTRY WHICH IMPEDE OR FACILITATE ADJUSTMENT

So far we have been considering adjustment factors in terms of the individual woman and her family. It is also important to note that a variety of factors external to her and her immediate kin have an effect. We have noted the effect of immigration classification upon access to services and employment. We now turn to other factors in the environment.

Attitudes of Members of the Dominant Culture

The attitudes of people in the new country are important in making the newcomer feel at home. Visible minorities are particularly at risk here. Racism and job discrimination are realities of life for black Canadians, and for Africans it is no different. Employment of black women in low positions is thought by some researchers to be more a problem of race than of gender (Estable, 1986; Ng, 1984; Ng and Gupta 1981). Boyd (1984) and Estable (1986) agree that all women immigrants are doubly disadvantaged because of their sex and countries of origin; however, when it comes to women of colour, the double disadvantage turns into triple jeopardy since they must "also face the pervasive racism of Canadian society" (Estable 1986, 23).

Historically, the lives of black people in North America have been characterized by slavery, oppression, and abject poverty. Tullock (1975, 140) feels that Canadian blacks, like their American counterparts, are victims of racism brought about by a legacy of slavery and its social and economic ramifications. A study of ethnic inequality and segregation in jobs in Toronto by Reitz, Calzavara, and Dasko (1981) found that women of West Indian origin were at the bottom of the wage scale, a fact that does not bode well for the African immigrant. In a study of fifty-two immigrant women employed in the domestic sector, Cohen (1987, 35) found that non-blacks were not employed in household jobs but 17 per cent of blacks were.

The members of the dominant culture may classify all blacks in the same group, but in fact Canadian blacks are from quite different cultural groups. Women from the Caribbean Islands form the majority of black immigrants in Canada. African immigrants, in contrast, come from many countries, speak different languages, belong to diverse religious groups, and have different cultural heritages. Whereas many Caribbean blacks come to Canada on work permits which specify low-status domestic work, Africans are not likely to do so and are instead likely to come under the family class. Since black immigrants from Africa so far have not aroused the curiosity of social scientists, we do not know how they are faring. We can expect that those who are disadvantaged in terms of language fluency or job status are treated like Caribbean blacks, who are subject to deplorable conditions, including racial discrimination, sexual exploitation, and invasion of privacy (Cohen 1987, 38).

Adaptation

When one combines the effects of the A factor (conditions associated with the stress of moving) with the B factor, (resources) and the C factor (interpretation of the host culture) all of which are affected by attitudes and policies of the dominant group, one can begin to predict X, adjustment. However, adjustment occurs over time, and here one must also account for the length of time in the new country.

Both Sluzki (1979) and Stein (1981) suggest that adjustment occurs in stages. At first, the newcomer experiences euphoria, particularly if she is a refugee and safe from the ravages of war. During this first rather short period, the person often sees the new country as a land of unlimited opportunity. Next, she needs to attend to her basic survival needs of food, clothing, and shelter, so that initially she may not pay attention to other needs. In the third and last phase, occurring three to five years after arrival, she is likely to feel discouraged. At this time, people may realize that their hopes and dreams of the new country may never be realized (Copeland and Harvey 1986).

DISCUSSION AND IMPLICATIONS

It is apparent that the lives of black immigrant women are characterized by stress arising in the workplace, the home, and the environment. Any institutional dynamics which underrate their skills and talent and deny them access to the services and occupations that are necessary for self-development hinder bonadaptation. As long as black immigrant women continue to experience hardships in terms of employment and language, and as long as they suffer discrimination on the basis of gender, sex, race, and even age, we can expect that their quality of life will be low.

We need research to understand the interplay of the variables used in immigrant adaptation. For example, if a woman has a good job, does this have a stronger influence than good health on her adjustment? What factors enable some people to adjust well in a subjective sense, even if objective conditions are poor? How do churches and religious beliefs contribute to or hinder bonadaptation? In what ways can family interaction overcome discrimination in the workplace? We think it is time for social scientists to stop overlooking the black African woman in Canada. We also think that using the double-ABCX model (McCubbin and Patterson 1983) can be most useful in understanding adaptation processes.

We also need to understand how black African women in Canada are helping themselves. For example there is an Immigrant Woman's Association in Manitoba, as well as a Manitoba chapter of the National Congress of Black Women. To what extent are these groups meeting the needs of black African immigrants? Are special associations of black African women available in all parts of the country, and are these associations pushing for political changes that will help their members? In addition to research on immigrant groups, helping professionals may assist in the development of ethnic networks to facilitate group interaction, which is helpful in itself and can also create political action.

Finally, policies and services of the dominant society have to be sensitive to the needs of these women. Black African women have to have adequate language training, available job training programs, good child care, and places where they can feel comfortable and make friends. Special efforts must be made to reach all sectors of the population (Burke 1984). We must not assume that current practices reach all immigrants equally, for they clearly do not.

It is our contention that black African women in Canada, like their sisters from other parts of the world, have survived and contributed to the society. What we need now are policies in place to facilitate bonadaptation and research to specify the exact conditions under which successful adjustment takes place.

REFERENCES

Arnopoulos, S.M. 1979. *Problems of Immigrant Women in the Canadian Labour Force*. Ottawa: Canadian Advisory Council on the Status of Women.

Bannerji, H., R. Ng, J. Scone, M. Silvera, and D. Khayatt 1987. "Immigrant Women in Canada: The Politics of Sex, Race and Class." *Resources for Feminist Research* 16: 3–4.

Bodner, A. and M. Reimer 1981. "The Organization of Social Services and Its Implications for Mental Health of Immigrant Women." In *By and About Immigrant Women*. Toronto: Cross-cultural Communications Centre.

Boss, P. 1970. "Family Stress." In M.B. Sussman and S.K. Steinmetz, eds., *Handbook of Marriage and the Family*. New York: Plenum Press.

Brody, E.B. 1970. *Behavior in a New Environment: Adaptations of Immigrant Populations*. Beverly Hills, California: Sage Publications.

Boyd, M. 1984. "At a Disadvantage: The Occupational Attainments of Foreign Born Women in Canada." *Journal of International Migration* 18: 10–91.

Bubolz, M.M., J.B. Eeicher, J.S. Evers, and S.M. Sontag 1980. "A Human Ecological Approach to Quality of Life: A Conceptual Framework and Results of a Preliminary Study." *Social Indicators Research* 7: 103–6.

Burk, M.E. 1984. "The Visible Minority Woman." *Currents* 1: 5–7.

Chan, K.B. and L. Lam 1983. "Resettlement of Vietnamese – Chinese Refugees in Montreal, Canada: Some Socio-psychological Problems and Dilemmas." *Canadian Ethnic Studies* 15: 1–17.

Cohen, R. 1987. "The Working Conditions of Immigrant Women: Live-in Domestics: Racism, Sexual Abuse and Invisibility." *Resources for Feminist Research* 16: 34–41.

Copeland, N. 1984. "Adaptation of Resettlement of Southeast Asian Adolescents." MA thesis, University of Manitoba, Winnipeg.

Copeland, N. and C.D.H. Harvey 1986. "Southeast Asians in Canada: Concern for Late Phases of Their Resettlement." *Canadian Home Economics Journal* 36: 111–13.

Copeland, N. and C.D.H. Harvey 1989. "Refugee Adaptation: The Case of Southeast Asian Youth in a Western Canadian City." *Canadian Home Economics Journal* 39: 163–7.

Estable, A. 1986. "Immigrant Women in Canada: Current Issues." Background paper prepared for the Canadian Advisory Council on the Status of Women, Ottawa.

Hill, R. 1949. *Families Under Stress*. New York: Harper and Row.

Huyck, E.E. and R. Fields 1981. "Impact of Resettlement on Refugee Children." *International Migration Review* 15: 246–54.

Manitoba. Employment Services and Economic Security 1983. "A Report on the Employment Status of Southeast Asian and Eastern European Immigrants."

McCubbin, H. and J.M. Patterson 1983. "Family Transitions: Adaptation to Stress." In H. McCubbin and C.R. Firley, eds., *Stress and the Family.* Vol. 1, *Coping with Normative Transitions,* 5–25. New York: Brunner/ Mazel.

Montero, D. 1979. *Vietnamese Americans: Patterns of Resettlement and Socioeconomic Adaptation in the U.S.A.* Boulder, Colorado: Westview Press.

Neuwirth, G. 1987. "The Socioeconomic Adjustment of Southeast Asian Refugees in Canada." Unpublished paper, University of Ottawa.

Ng, R. 1984. "Immigrant Women and the State." PHD thesis, Ontario Institute for Studies in Education, Toronto.

Ng, R. and D. Gupta 1981. "Nation Builders? The Captive Labour Force of the Non-English Speaking Immigrant Woman." *Canadian Women's Studies* 3: 83–85.

Reitz, J., L. Calzavara, and D. Dasko 1981. "Discrimination or Adjustment? Visible Minority Women in the Labour Force." *Currents* 1: 28–30.

Richmond, A.H. 1974. "Aspects of the Absorption and Adaptation of Immigrants." On file, Employment and Immigration Canada, Ottawa.

Richmond, A.H. 1984. "Socio-cultural Adaptation and Conflict in Immigrant Receiving Countries." *International Social Science Journal* 36: 519–36.

Rogers, W.L. and P.E. Converse 1975. "Measures of the Perceived Overall Quality of Life." *Social Indicators Research* 2: 127–52.

Samuel, T.J. 1984. "Economic Adaptation of Refugees in Canada: Experience of an Earlier Century." *International Migration Review* 22: 45–54.

Sluzki, C.E. 1979. "Migration and Family Conflict." *Family Process* 18: 379–90.

Stein, B. 1981. "The Refugee Experience: Defining the Parameters of a Field of Study." *International Migration Review* 15: 320–30.

Taft, R. and R. Johnson 1967. "The Assimilation of Adolescent Polish Immigrants and Parent – Child Interation." *Merrill-Palmer Quarterly* 13: 111–20.

Tullock, H. 1975. *Black Canadians: A Long Line of Fighters.* Toronto: NC Press.

MONIQUE RAIMBAULT

Women with Disabilities: A Research Survey Report[1]

This research survey completes a two-phase project on the effects of being female and disabled on economic independence. A fifty-six question survey, administered in January 1987 to 757 disabled women living in both urban and rural Manitoba, provided research materials on a severely under-represented group whose voice has rarely been heard from a research perspective. This has been one of the first times that disabled women's ideas and opinions have been not only documented but collected with the purpose of following through and acting upon these identified ideas and themes. By gaining insight into the daily realities of women with disabilities, we will have a greater understanding of how the women's movement can better serve them in the formation and execution of feminist policy.

Femmes handicapées: rapport d'un sondage

Ce sondage de recherche complète un projet en deux étapes sur les conséquences pour l'autonomie financière du fait d'être femme et handicapée. Un sondage de 56 questions distribué en janvier 1987 à 757 femmes handicapées vivant en milieu rural et urbain, au Manitoba, a fourni des données de recherche sur un groupe fortement sous-représenté auquel on demande rarement de se faire entendre. C'est l'une des premières occasions où les idées et les opinions des femmes handicapées ont été non seulement documentées mais aussi recueillies dans le but d'y donner suite. Un aperçu des réalités quotidiennes des femmes handicapées, nous fera mieux comprendre comment le mouvement des femmes peut les aider davantage dans l'élaboration et la mise en oeuvre d'une politique féministe.

INTRODUCTION

The Consulting Committee on the Status of Women with Disabilities (CCSWD) was established in 1984 to forge links between the movement for disabled consumers and the women's movement and to better address the needs and concerns of women with disabilities. It was agreed that, to gain a better understanding of the double jeopardy faced by women with disabilities, research must first be conducted. Thus the Department of the Secretary of State was approached for research funding to document the social and economic needs and strengths of women with disabilities.

The research proposal was divided into two phases. The first, undertaken from February to June 1986, involved a comprehensive literature review, personal interviews with thirty-two participants, and the construction of a questionnaire design. The second phase, running for five months starting in December 1986, saw the actual administration of the survey questionnaire to 757 disabled women living in Manitoba, followed by data analysis and summation in a final report.

The objectives of the research project included gaining a better understanding of the effects on economic independence of being female and disabled, as well as discovering what resources women with disabilities need to improve their economic independence and other aspects of their social condition. The survey gave us a good basis for a profile of disabled women living in Manitoba. It has also yielded an understanding of employment patterns and conditions for women with disabilities and the relationship of disability to economic security. The numerical data gathered from the survey have been complemented by the personal interviews, which provided more qualitative information. This paper discusses the research methods and sample frame used for the survey and includes data analysis along with interpretations. It culminates in a summary and conclusions.

The project has provided one of the first opportunities not only for the documentation of disabled women's ideas and opinions but also for collecting these views for the purpose of acting upon the identified ideas and themes. In fact, few research projects have dealt specifically with disabled women.

This population deserves far more political and social attention, not only to uncover the structural inequalities women with disabilities face but also to discover the unique gifts they have to offer women's groups, the disabled community, and society at large. The dissemination of the following information should have far-reaching effects for both the movement for disabled consumers and the women's movement, but most importantly for disabled women themselves. We need to access this community, for they are a powerful group of women whose voice must be heard.

STUDY DESIGN

Sampling Frame

Our target population, women with physical disabilities of mobility, hearing, or sight,[2] was sampled in two stages. The first stage, held in May 1986, consisted of personal interviews with thirty-two participants. Through snowball sampling with contacts obtained from various disability organizations, we secured the names of approximately forty women who might be interested in being interviewed.

This was not a representative sample; the women were not assessed for age, income, or other factors because of the time limitations of the project and the difficulty in securing names. The four trained interviewers generally reported positive encounters with participants. The women were for the most part very open and eager to share opinions and experiences.[3]

Sampling Method

The second stage included a systematic non-probability sample of women registered with various disability organizations in the city of Winnipeg. An approximate number of female members aged 16–65 from twenty-one disability groups was obtained to get an idea of population size. We identified a total of 6,741 Manitoba women with disabilities, and we decided to sample 15% of this population, or 1,011 women. In order to obtain as random a sample as possible, we asked the disability groups to send questionnaires to approximately every seventh female on their membership list.

DATA ANALYSIS

The survey objectives included creating a profile of disabled women living in Manitoba (*see* Table 1) and collecting data on the effects of being both female and disabled on economic independence. Data analysis will be divided into seven survey categories culminating in a summary of findings, thus providing us with a better understanding of the effects of the double jeopardy faced by women with disabilities.

Table 1
Profile of Respondents

Average age (years)	28
Age at onset of disability (percent)	
Congenital	36
Acquired between ages 20 and 39	21
Disability type	
Mobility impaired	26%
Agility impaired	34%
Visually impaired	20%
Hearing impaired	20%
Educational level (some or completed)	
High school	45%
Post-secondary education	38%
University	19%
Unemployment rate	69%
Average income	
Personal	$6,015
Household[1]	$14,719
Marital and family status	
Single	44%
Married or common law	39%
Separated or divorced	10%
With children	46%
Age of disability onset and marital status	
Onset before age 15	67% single[2]
Onset age 15–65	18% single

[1] 60% living with family or spouse

[2] Women whose disability occurred before age nineteen are three times less likely to have children than those whose disability began later.

Education

This section dealt with the educational levels attained by women with disabilities, as education has long been viewed as one of the avenues of advancement in society. Of the respondents aged 25 to 34, 58% had up to grade 12 and 19% had university or graduate studies, with an equal number enrolled in community college. Compared with information tables from Statistics Canada, levels of education do not differ significantly for disabled Manitoban women and average Canadian women. Of the average Canadian female aged 25 to 34, 59% had up to grade 12 and 41% had some postsecondary education including community college, compared to our total of 38%.

If the assumption that disabled women are less educated than ablebodied women holds true, then our survey reached a more

highly educated portion of the disabled female population. The
survey sampled a large number of women who are either presently
enrolled in post-secondary education or have obtained degrees.
These women may have a better understanding of the purpose and
usefulness of surveys and therefore may complete them more readily
than disabled women living alone and isolated from mainstream
society.

Our most significant finding was that those who attended special
schools for the disabled had lower-than-average figures for educational attainment. It would thus seem this population is ill-prepared
for furthering their studies, especially since none of the women
surveyed who had attended special schools entered university.

Comparing age at onset of disability to level of education revealed
that the level of education was significantly lowest when the disability
first occured between the ages of 11 and 14. Other age groups did
not demonstrate a markable relationship. It thus seems that disability
occurring at this age level greatly affects the respondents' future
attainments.

Employment

Statistics Canada concludes "the higher an individual's level of education, the greater the chance of that person being part of the
labour force." (Statistics Canada 1985*a*, 26). Therefore educational
achievement may have great bearing on economic independence as
it supposedly leads to greater employment opportunities.

Data on finances and employment were important to our study,
since we hoped to assess the economic independence of women with
disabilities. According to this survey, 69% of the respondents are
unemployed, compared to Statistics Canada's figure of 7.7% for
Manitoban women as a group (Statistics Canada 1985*b*, 64). The
employment figure gathered from this survey (29%) corresponds
closely to that reported in a study of northwestern Ontario, which
found that 30% of the disabled women in Thunder Bay were employed (Ontario March of Dimes 1985).

Before discussing the financial realities of women with disabilities,
we should explore the barriers that disabled women perceive as
preventing them from finding and maintaining employment. Of the
women who answered the question, an astonishing 73% cited lack
of training as the barrier to their finding employment. This is a key
question in the study of economic independence and women with
disabilities, as this is the very reason stated as responsible for their
economic dependence.

Income

The main source of income of Manitoba women with disabilities is social assistance (24%), closely followed by support from family or friends (20%) and employment wages (20%). Though 29% of the respondents are presently employed, only 20% are able to support themselves on their wages. The average personal income of the 165 who responded to this question was $6,015 per year. Statistics Canada's figure of average earnings for Manitoba women (1985a) was $11,655. Therefore, according to the survey, disabled women are earning 90% of the earnings of the average Manitoba female, who in turn earns 56% of the earnings of the average Manitoba male (1985 figures).

The population surveyed is relatively well-educated compared to the average Canadian female. It can be assumed that education leads to greater employment opportunities; however, despite their education, 69% of the respondents are nevertheless unemployed.

Medical

Several questions on medical issues were included, since recent literature on women with disabilities suggests this population faces particular difficulties in dealing with the health care profession.

Questions on health issues yielded surprisingly positive results from the survey. Of those questioned, 71% stated that they had adequate medical knowledge about their disability, and 72% stated their present medical facilities were meeting their needs. A possible explanation for these high statistics is that disabled women registered with consumer organizations may be better integrated into society and are therefore in a better position to demand proper health care.

We can safely say that very little research deals with the medical concerns of women with disabilities, and some respondents noted that education is needed for both women *and* the medical profession on this group's health care needs.

Housing

This section hoped to gain an idea of housing needs and present arrangements for women with disabilities. It was interesting to note that 35% of the respondents lived with a spouse (or equivalent); 25% lived with parents and family, and 29% lived on their own. Most women indicated satisfaction with present housing arrangements regardless of housing situation, be it family unit, apartment with support services, or another alternative.

The "Social Needs Assessment Study," sponsored by the Manitoba League of the Physically Handicapped, states that "single, and female individuals experience the greatest difficulties in the attainment of a more independent lifestyle (Manitoba League of the Physically Handicapped 1984). The little literature that does exist on disabled women and housing needs refers mostly to problems encountered in nursing homes.

Many women mentioned the frustration of living in a physically inaccessible house and expressed the need to do such things as build ramps or install visual door bells. Because of economic realities, alternatives are not easily accessible to them. As one middle-aged woman stated, "The upkeep, taxes, and so on ... without employment make it difficult. The real issue here is the unemployment factor."

Relationships and women with disability issues

Of the respondents, 80% stated they had fulfilling personal relationships, people with whom they can discuss personal matters. It would thus appear that maintaining close friendships was not problematic for the women surveyed. Fifty-four percent stated that they did not feel isolated or alone. However, they seemed to need to meet more women in similar situations, since 54% stated they would indeed like the opportunity to meet more women with disabilities.

One interesting point was the differences in response to questions on whether the women's movement has improved the general situation of women and whether it has helped improve the respondent's personal life. Forty-seven percent stated the women's movement has improved the general situation of women and only 22% felt it had personally improved their life. A further 32% flatly disagreed that the women's movement had personally benefited them. These questions also had one of the highest response rates in the questionnaire. A possible conclusion drawn from these statistics is that women with disabilities are not well served by the women's movement.

SUMMARY AND CONCLUSIONS

Survey results and analysis gathered from the research project have advanced the basic understanding of disabled women's social reality. By documenting and quantifying daily realities faced by women with disabilities, it helps to identify common threads and social problems. What may be perceived as a personal problem can now be seen as a social problem or condition when we see that certain issues affect many women with disabilities. Personal issues then become political ones. Certain patterns emerge when we conduct social research; these patterns lead to a greater understanding of the double jeopardy faced by women with disabilities.

The logic used to move from empirical data to descriptive analysis is carefully described in the report, and results have led to a greater appreciation of the difficulty disabled women have in maintaining economic security. The research project has discovered and brought to light the economic reality of women with disabilities, in particular their rate of unemployment and the paucity of job opportunities existing for this population. Though the women surveyed are relatively well educated, their income is well below the poverty line and very few actually hold down paying jobs.

The survey generated strong emotion among respondents. Some were offended by the questionnaire, deeming it far too personal. One woman expressed outrage saying, "Let me ask you one question; would you send this to an able-bodied woman and expect her to answer it? It's things like this questionnaire that make me realize just how uneducated you people really are about disabled women." Others expressed concern and confusion about segregating disabled people, but for the most part respondents made positive remarks about the survey. As one woman said, "I really appreciated filling out the survey, not only because it might help other women with disabilities, but also because it gives me a chance to see myself a little more clearly."

Data analysis shows a need for disabled women to organize, emphasizing educational activities for both disabled women and the general public. We need ongoing research projects to explore further issues brought to light by this research, and we must create support networks and social activities for women with disabilities.

Manitoba was in need of research materials which study the effects of being female and disabled on economic independence. Although disabled women of Manitoba experience particular economic and social realities as Manitobans, all disabled women across Canada share similar concerns by virtue of their double jeopardy. This sense of solidarity, in conjunction with community organizing in all provinces, will inevitably lead to greater social opportunities, increased independence, and (most importantly) the removal of barriers impeding disabled women's control over their lives.

NOTES

1 This study was sponsored by the Consulting Committee on the Status of Women with Disabilities (CCSWD).
2 While it is in solidarity with mentally handicapped women's needs and concerns, the CCSWD does not address this group of women because their history and social problems differ significantly from those of physically disabled women.
3 For a detailed report of the first phase of research, please consult the "Research Project Report on Women with Disabilities 1986," available from the CCSWD.

REFERENCES

Ontario March of Dimes 1985. *Women and Disabilities: Life in Northwestern Ontario*. Thunder Bay: Ontario March of Dimes.
Manitoba League of the Physically Handicapped. "Social Needs Assessment Study." Report on file.
Statistics Canada 1985a. *Women in Canada: A Statistical Report*. Ottawa: Statistics Canada. Catalogue number 89–503.
Statistics Canada 1985b. *The Labour Force*. Ottawa: Statistics Canada. Catalogue number 71–001.

MARY O'BRIEN

Never-Married Older Women: Beyond the Stereotypes[1]

Many stereotypes influence attitudes toward never-married women. There is very little existing data on their actual life experiences and how they have handled singlehood over a lifetime. In addition, we do not know if they are subject to some of the common stereotypes of old age. This paper examines and analyses these issues by reporting on in-depth interviews with fifteen never-married women who were 80 years of age and over. Although we found a great diversity, most of these women had satisfying relationships with family members and friends and were able to handle the constraints of age positively and realistically.

Les célibataires âgées: au delà des stéréotypes

Une foule de stéréotypes influencent les attitudes à l'endroit des femmes célibataires. Nous ne disposons que de très peu de données sur leurs expériences de vie réelles et sur leur manière d'assumer leur célibat tout au long de leur vie. En outre, nous ignorons si elles sont touchées par certains stéréotypes répandus relatifs à l'âge avancé. Cet article étudie ces questions et en fait l'analyse en faisant un compte-rendu d'entrevues en profondeur avec quinze femmes de quatre-vingts ans et plus qui ont toujours été célibataires. Bien qu'on ait relevé une grande diversité, ces femmes ont entretenu des relations satisfaisantes avec les membres de leur famille et leurs relations d'amitié, et elles ont été en mesure de faire face d'une manière positive et réaliste aux diminutions qui accompagnent le vieillissement.

INTRODUCTION

Until recently, never-married people have been included with the widowed, separated, and divorced in research studies. Only in the past few years have they become the focus of research as an independent group, and as that focus emerges, gender and age have not been accounted for. As interest grows in older never-marrieds, particularly never-married *women*, we are finding more information on gender difference (Braito and Anderson 1984).

Currently, however, there is very little data on the life experiences of never-married older women, and many questions have yet to be addressed. Are they subject to some of the common stereotypes of old age in addition to those associated with being never married? How have they coped with singlehood over a lifetime? How have they handled life changes and the aging process?

To explore these questions, in-depth interviews were conducted with fifteen never-married women, 80 years and over, living in community settings in Prince Edward Island. Prince Edward Island is unique in that it has both the highest proportion of the elderly (12.5 per cent compared to the national rate of 10 per cent) and of never-married women over 75 (15 per cent of the elderly, according to the 1981 Census). The study had three purposes: to identify the personal, social, and economic factors which might influence the never-married older woman's ability to deal with everyday living and the changes that occur with aging; to evaluate some of the common stereotypes of never-marrieds; and to identify the specific needs of this group as an aid to developing appropriate social policies.

METHODOLOGY

The survey used a qualitative approach in order to incorporate the participants' understanding and interpretation of the decision-making processes, life events, and conflicts which shaped their lives. Furthermore, this approach allowed for examination of the attitudes and assumptions which lie behind those processes. An initial questionnaire helped to gather demographic data. During the following three or four interviews of an hour each, each interviewee answered open-ended questions that reviewed various phases of her life. Transcripts of the open-ended interviews were examined and the following categories were selected for data analysis: reflections and views on childhood; family and community relationships; career development and work life; self-perceptions as a person and as a single woman; problems and satisfactions experienced; and adjustments to life-changes and the experience of aging.

STUDY FINDINGS

About half of the women who were interviewed were between eighty and eighty-five years of age and the remainder were between eighty-six and ninety. The majority were living alone in their own houses and apartments in one of the two main urban centers on the island. All but one had spent her childhood and early youth in Price Edward Island and half had grown up in rural areas of the province. Most had come from large families and maintained strong family ties. There was no particular pattern in birth order. While health and mobility problems were common – about half needed help with shopping and transportation – most of the women considered themselves better off than their peers. Nearly all were satisfied with their friendships and with family relationships in general.

The women who participated in the study came from a broad range of family backgrounds and living situations, yet the similarities in their perceptions of their formative years are more striking than the differences.

The general image of childhood, as they saw it, is one of security, harmonious family life with a clear separation of parental roles, certainty and acceptance of rules and social norms, and a strong sense of belonging to one's community. Perhaps the most frequent impression of childhood that was conveyed was one of being well taken care of by good parents, of a secure, harmonious, close family life. "I had a really lovely childhood. My parents were marvelous. I always remember that sort of warmth and assurance that I got from my father and mother."

Mothers' roles were quite distinct and well-defined in the families of these women. The household was clearly the mother's domain. Several of the women expressed strong admiration and affection for their fathers. Participants differed somewhat on which parent was seen as the authority figure in the household. Some could clearly point to their mothers as the disciplinarian; others saw father as the boss. Relationships with brothers and sisters were usually described as harmonious, especially in the large, rural families. There were some hints of sisterly conflict – "sister was mother's favourite ... sister didn't share the housework" – but all seemed to get along with brothers. None of the women expressed any strong feelings of discrimination against girls in the family; if it occurred, it was accepted or went unnoticed. It is interesting to note that some respondents perceived their brothers as more adventuresome and independent than they, and some noted that their brothers would occasionally resist parental authority whereas they would not.

As is typical of never-married women, the women in this study were relatively well educated for their generation (Spreitzer and Riley 1974). The majority had initially completed high school and more than half had some post-secondary education; three of these had bachelor's degrees and two master's degrees. "School was a happy place for me. I liked it; I enjoyed it. I loved it. I wanted to get an education, which I did. I got through for a teacher." Some recalled the importance of good education to them and to their parents. In rural areas, the mother was more often mentioned as the parent who encouraged education. "Mother would have liked all of us to have gone to university. But dad, it didn't seem to matter to him one way or the other."

University education was a rare thing for girls and the only degree-granting college on the island did not accept females. Some of the women spoke of the rarity of anyone leaving the rural community to continue her education. They were often the only ones in their age group to do so and sometimes the only members of their family. Some continued their education during their working careers, sometimes taking time off from work, sometimes attending summer schools, until they reached their objectives.

Career options for young women, as perceived by the study participants, were very few in the early decades of the century. Apart from the limited options open to young women at the time, perhaps the most striking aspect of early career goals and choices was the influence of the family. A strong sense of obligation to the family could result in educational and career goals being postponed for a number of years. One woman, whose family could not afford to send her to university, delayed her education until she was no longer needed at home. Another postponed her early ambition of leaving Prince Edward Island to teach elsewhere in Canada until both her parents had died. Family ties and obligations remained strong throughout their working lives for nearly all of the women; two returned to the island in mid-life because their families needed them.

Although some of the study participants spoke of goals they had set early in life, few of the women had strong career plans that they followed consistently. Career interests and ambitions seemed instead to evolve as they matured and were often quite circumstantial. What seemed to carry most of them through their careers was not ambition but a desire to do well at what they were doing and to be helpful and useful to others. "I always enjoyed teaching, and I felt that I helped somebody in my work. That was rewarding." Their occupations were varied; the participants included teachers, nurses, one self-employed businesswoman, a companion, and a supervisor in a utility company. One woman stayed on the family farm all of her life and another had devoted most of her career to volunteer community work.

A final observation on career goals that emerges from the interviews is that their plans were likely to remain tentative and short-term as long as marriage remained a possibility. Some women appeared to postpone career plans until their status as single women was established and accepted. Thus, as the women matured, new interests and ambitions often evolved.

However, work did become an important part of the women's lives, both as a source of income and as a means of achieving a positive self-identity. There was much evidence of a strong work commitment among the women. For one woman, teaching became "the love of my life," and she further stated, "they couldn't pry me loose with a stick." It was also important to most of these women to know that they were doing their jobs well. A woman who set up her own business, in which she was very successful, spoke frequently of her lifelong commitment to hard work. "Oh, I always worked ... my business was working ... all my life ... Today I could make a fortune if I was 20 years younger and able to work. It makes me sick that I can't work." Some of the women showed a strong interest in advancement in their jobs or professions, another indication of strong work commitment. More than half of the working women attained positions of responsibility in which they were supervising others or training other professionals.

Considering that most of the study participants achieved satisfaction in their working lives, it is interesting to note that many found their early work experiences very difficult and stressful. They resolved their difficulties with work in different ways: by a complete change of work, by advancement to a higher level in their professions, or, in the case of a woman who found teaching difficult, by "sticking it out" and, after a few years, learning to love it.

Job changes were frequent for many of the women. A sense of adventure seems to have prompted others to change careers. Two went overseas during World War II, one as a nurse, one as a Red Cross worker. Another, who had taught school for several years, went to western Canada to work in the hotel business when the opportunity presented itself. It seems clear from their comments that these women were community-minded for most of their lives, usually holding executive positions in voluntary organizations.

It has been suggested that the loss of work role is more problematic for never-married persons than for the married (Ward 1979). The transition from career to retirement was a difficult one for most of these women. During this time they had experienced a deep sense of loss. "I really didn't feel that I should retire, I felt that I have a lot to give." "I thought, 'What good am I? Nobody wants me, nobody needs me; I'm not working, I'm no good to anybody.' I had that awful feeling ... but I got over it." Typically, they substituted other activities and relationships for those lost with retirement. Some became more active in volunteer work and community organizations in which they had previously participated. Others started a number of new activities. By being joiners they not only fulfilled their need to be useful to others but also met needs for social activity and status in the community.

Three aspects of the participants' lives as single women were examined in this study: perceptions and recollections of why they did not marry; the difficulties they experienced as single women; and feelings about on-the-job discrimination toward women.

None of the women who were interviewed said that at any point in their lives they made a conscious decision not to marry. Nor did marriage appear to be an important goal in any of their lives. Most had friendships with men and opportunities to marry, but seemed to be very hesitant about relinquishing their independence. "As a young teenager, I always believed in women's lib ... I wouldn't take the vow to obey that used to be in the marriage ceremony." "A lot of people just get married. But there was no point in me doing that; it would just be a burden on me to marry anyone I wasn't really in love with ... I'm sort of like a plant. I want to grow in my own way."

Other women said that they had not met the right person or that marriage was not one of their goals. One woman's comment – that it was pretty hard for an independent woman to make marriage work – sums up the attitudes of the majority. What seems to have happened is that as time went on, the marriage question merely decreased in importance as an issue in their lives. As midlife approached, most of them were otherwise involved in career or community work or both.

The question of difficulties as a single woman seemed to be almost an irrelevant one. If single life was a disadvantage, study participants were unaware of it. They were absorbed in their careers and in community activities, and enjoyed friendships with other single women. While no one found single life a difficult state, five of the women expressed regret at not having had children, but once again some women considered the difficulties and confinements of marriage to be not enough of a tradeoff for the joys of parenthood.

Most of the women interviewed had entered women's professions. This may be one reason why job discrimination was not an issue for most of them in their working careers. Their comments indicate, however, that they did not feel discrimination as women because they accepted as normal the constraints of few career options and lower pay for women. Only two of the women said that they had ever been aware of receiving lower pay than men for similar work. It had not occurred to either of them to object to this.

While most of the women were not aware of any discrimination against them as women, some had mixed feelings about the feminist movement but were hopeful for change. "Eventually women can be independent and men can be independent and still admire each other. I think women should be treated equally but I don't believe in being militant about it. It's understanding that brings people together."

Some insight was gained into the personalities and attitudes of the study participants when they were asked what motivating forces guided them and how they handled difficult times. Most of the interviewees felt that they had, in their lives, let nature take its course. As one woman put it, "I went along with life." Some of the group were clearly risk-takers, making moves and job changes which must have required courage. Others were fighters; they had pulled themselves through difficult periods by sheer determination. Other women clearly saw themselves as "doers" who had played an active role in shaping their lives and the lives of others. The women in this group seemed determined to do well at their jobs, to achieve, and to bring about change where they saw change was needed. This determination may have been the strong motivating force which guided their lives. The study participants as a whole, believed life motivation and the inner strength to deal with difficulties came mainly from the values instilled by their parents and families or from their religious beliefs.

And finally, here is one woman's philosophy on dealing with failure: "A failure is difficult. You have to adjust to that, and you can't win every time, you know. Somebody else is going to win sometimes and you have to adjust to that. If you have a few aspects of your life that you're successful in, you're lucky."

The need to be useful and to help others came out in some of their expressed hopes for the future. For one woman, this wish took precedence over any thoughts of disability or dependency. "I hope that I can be of some use in the world and that I can have a little bit of influence in alleviating the terrific amount of suffering that there is in the world today. Those are the only things that really matter, to make life better for other people."

Most accepted the limitations of advancing age realistically. Looking back with regret did not appear to be a preoccupation with these women. While some conceded they would do a few things differently if they had their lives to live over, it was not something they spent a lot of time worrying about.

While the literature suggests that most older unmarried people rely primarily on community supports (Kivett and Learner 1980), one important finding that emerges from the interviews and from the impressions of the interviewers is that most of the women had strong support networks of family and friends. All respondents had at least one important friend. Some had compensated for losses of age peers by making friends with younger women. The majority mentioned nieces, nephews, brothers, and sisters as important in their lives. They dealt with restrictions on physical mobility by accepting more help from family and friends. Their strong sense of connection and belonging to the island seemed to offer a certain kind of security in their old age.

CONCLUSIONS

Much available research about never-married persons suggests the following: that never-marrieds of both genders have had poor family relationships (Spreitzer and Riley 1974); that their inadequacies stereotype them as losers (Stein 1976); that older never-marrieds constitute a special social type in that they have been lifelong loners and live more isolated lives (Gubrium 1976); that they have difficulty living in a world where marriage is the norm (Edwards and Hoover 1974); and that in old age they have more problematic lives and are less happy than married persons due to lack of family ties and intimate relationships (Ward 1979). Admittedly, participants in this study represent a select group, a fact which probably accounts for the high levels of life satisfaction reported. However none of the generalizations just mentioned describes the women in this study. These women were able to substitute available satisfactions for losses incurred and to ask for help when help was needed. Some women showed conscious suppression of problems and a control of negative feelings, but these can be considered realistic, positive, and rational ways of adjusting to age-related changes (Butler and Lewis 1982). As we study future cohorts of never-married women, researchers need to keep in mind the diversity that exists within this group. As Rubinstein (1987) reminds us, cultural traditions, family orientations, personalities and personal ambitions, sexual preferences, and even demographic factors affect all elderly persons, regardless of marital status.

One of the greatest needs that never-married women have is for more formal support in later life. Although nearly all of the women had accepted increasing dependence on others in their present lives, it is unlikely that family and friends could be relied upon for help in the event that more caregiving was needed in the future. As is true elsewhere, such support would not likely be forthcoming (Johnson and Catalano 1981). Even though family traditions and ties in

Prince Edward Island are considered strong and are still governed by such basic values as family obligation and family loyalty, these and other values are in a state of transition. More than 7 per cent of Prince Edward Island's elderly live in government manors or private nursing homes (Prince Edward Island Department of Health and Social Services 1981). Most of these persons are never married, widowed, or divorced (Statistics Canada 1981). Perhaps more important are the attitude of the women themselves. Only one woman in this study mentioned moving in with relatives as an alternative offered in the event of her becoming unable to live on her own. Her reasons for rejecting this offer reflect the feelings of many older persons – she wished to maintain the independence she valued so highly. Independent living was necessary for these women to maintain their psychological integrity. For women who have remained single, the maintenance of personal dignity and positive self-image in their later years consists in retaining the kind of control over their life decisions that they have developed and cherished over a lifetime. With more women opting for singlehood, it is reasonable to assume that their numbers will increase. Today's never-married older women may be able to shed light on future concerns and needs. For instance, what kinds of supports, both formal and informal, can realistically abate rates of institutionalization for these women and for those who are widowed and have no children?

At the same time, older women who never married can serve as role models for today's younger women who, regardless of marital status, are striving for autonomy and identities apart from traditional roles. Many have been in unique positions in that they have not derived their social standing from men but have found it necessary to build their own identities through personal and professional achievement. Certainly these women are examples of courage and resourcefulness.

By inviting them to tell their stories we can also glean some advice about resisting the mania to remain young with the knowledge that a rich life can await us as we age. Never-married older women's strong sense of independence can give some insights into what the future can look like for today's younger women. And as more and more women live into their eighties and nineties, it becomes increasingly important that their experience of the aging process and old age be better understood for the sake of correcting stereotypes and setting forth models of successful aging. The lives of these women need to be made more visible.

NOTES

1 This article originally appeared in *Canadian Woman Studies/les cahiers de la femme* 8(4): 77–80 (Winter 1987). This research project was funded by CRIAW, The Social Science Research Council of Canada, and the Department of Secretary of State. Francis Piercey and Olive Bryanton helped with the data collection and analysis for this study.

REFERENCES

Braito, R. and D. Anderson 1984. "The Ever-Single Elderly Woman." In E. Markson, ed., *Older Women: Issues and Prospects*. Markson, Toronto: Lexington Press, 195–225.

Butler, R. and M. Lewis 1982. *Aging and Mental Health: Positive Psychosocial and Biomedical Approaches*. St. Louis: C.V. Mosby.

Edwards, M. and E. Hoover 1974. *The Challenge of Being Single in Old Age*. Los Angeles: J.P. Tarcher.

Gubrium, J. 1976. "Being Single in Old Age." In J. Gubrium, ed., *Time, Roles and Self in Old Age*. New York: Human Science Press.

Johnson, C. and D. Catalano 1981. "Childless Elderly and Their Supports." *The Gerontologist* 21: 610–18.

Kivett, V. and R. Learner 1980. "Perspectives on the Childless Rural Elderly: A Comparative Analysis." *The Gerontologist* 20: 708–16.

Prince Edward Island. Department of Social Services 1981. *Towards Meeting the Needs of Senior Citizens in P.E.I.* Charlottetown: Department of Social Services.

Rubinstein, R. 1987. "Never Married as Social Type: Re-evaluating Some Images." *The Gerontologist* 27: 108–13.

Spreitzer. E. and L. Riley 1974. "Factors Associated with Singlehood." *Journal of Marriage and the Family* 36: 533–42.

Statistics Canada 1982. "Age, Sex and Marital Status." 1981 Census of Canada.

Statistics Canada 1984. *The Elderly in Canada*. (1981 census) Ottawa: Minister of Supply and Services, April.

Stein, P. 1976. *Single*. Englewood Cliffs, N.J.: Prentice Hall.

Ward, R. 1979. "Never Married in Later Life." *Journal of Gerontology* 34: 861–69.

MADELINE JEAN GRAVELINE

Threats to Rural Women's Well-Being: A Group Response

For those living outside of major urban centers, rural life has both challenges and satisfactions. One well-known difficulty is the limited availability of services, particularly mental health services. Women, who make up a large percentage of our clients, are challenged by economic, political, and personal invisibility. Some of the contributing factors include: underemployment; lack of child care, public transportation, and educational opportunities; limited political representation; time constraints; and isolation due to geographical distance and the conservative milieu. Feminist support and action groups are explored as a successful strategy to provide an opportunity for connection and empowerment of rural women personally and politically.

Une réaction collective aux obstacles au bien-être des femmes vivant à la campagne

Vivre dans un milieu rural apporte à la fois des satisfactions et des défis. Un des problèmes bien connus est le manque de services, notamment dans le domaine de la santé mentale. Les femmes, qui constituent une partie importante de notre clientèle, sont aux prises avec le manque de visibilité sur les plans économique, politique et personnel, dont les causes sont notamment le sous-emploi, la pénurie des services de garde, de transport en commun et des possibilités d'éducation, une représentation politique restreinte, le manque de temps, et l'isolement dû à l'éloignement géographique et au milieu conservateur. On étudie la possibilité de faire appel aux groupes de soutien et d'action féministes pour que les femmes vivant en milieu rural puissent établir des contacts et gagner du pouvoir sur les plans personnel et politique.

The oppression of women in Canada today is a well-documented reality (Fitzgerald, Guberman, and Wolfe 1982; Turner and Emery 1983). We are defined as inferior to men, and this presumed inferiority is then used as an explanation and rationalization for the denial of equal access to society's opportunities. Women's oppression is reinforced by the sense of helplessness created by this situation. This may translate into behaviour which suggests lack of confidence, ability, or capacity to affect changes in ourselves or in the systems that victimize us (Norman and Mancuso 1980). This lack of personal power is reflected in the large number of women who use mental health services (Smith and David 1975).

This paper examines the lives of rural women, focusing both on women as individuals, struggling with personal problems, and women as a social group, pressured and pigeon-holed by social structures and institutions. We will look beyond the threats to well-being inherent in rural society and explore the opportunity for promoting wellness available in all-woman support and action groups.

An initial clarification of the term "rural" is in order, particularly in a province like Manitoba, where over 50 per cent of the population lives in one urban center. "Rural women" can refer to Third World women, farm women, women in single-resource communities, or small-town women. For the purposes of this paper the term "rural woman" will refer to women outside major Canadian urban centers. The specific issues of farm women and single-resource community women will be acknowledged.

Considering the paucity of information regarding rural women, it seems safe to assume that an overall characteristic of this group is its invisibility. While invisibility may pervade all areas, three will be highlighted: economic, political, and personal power.

The economic plight of women has been well researched (Armstrong and Armstrong 1982; O'Connell 1983). Three out of five poor adults in Canada are women. According to the report "Women and Poverty" (1979), being a poor woman is directly connected to the assumption that women will take on the bulk of the responsibility for raising the children and maintaining the home, while men provide the financial security. Because of this assumption, women are improperly trained for paid jobs and are denied access to better positions with advancement opportunities.

The economic recession in the 1980s has created an atmosphere of instability in rural areas since farms and small businesses are going bankrupt and main industries are closing. Women in record numbers are seeking employment to help stabilize the family finances. A recent study of sixty rural women in Manitoba indicated that

81.7 per cent were employed full-time or part-time in the family business or community (Potter and Dustan 1983). Eichler (1983) indicates that this rural trend is in keeping with overall Canadian employment statistics.

For most women, accepting paid employment means carrying two fulltime jobs. The "average" Canadian woman employed outside the home does approximately 30 to 35 hours per week of housework and child care (Manitoba Department of Labour 1981). Farm wives put in a good deal of unpaid farm labour – 20 to 40 hours per week between May and November and 33.8 hours per week between December and April (Saskatchewan Labour 1981). Men, on the other hand, were found to increase their housework and childcare contributions by an average of 1 hour per week when their partners took jobs outside the home (Meissner and Humpreys 1975; Clark and Harvey 1976).

These figures support the major complaint of rural women brought out in the Ontario Study on Rural Women (McGhee 1984), namely time constraints and heavy workloads.

For women who work outside the home, the lack of child care in rural areas is a major problem. Today, very few extended family members live nearby, and if they do they are often in the work force themselves. Lack of affordable and accessible child care not only curtails women's necessary involvement in the paid labour force, but it may also limit the training opportunities they need for advancement. In the Ontario study previously cited (McGhee 1984), women noted that many job training and retraining courses are offered in urban centres and are often inaccessible because of distance. Unless a woman can prove to funders that she is a main contributor to the family income (difficult when she often gets little or no pay for much of her work), she is ineligible for an allowance to cover child care expenses. Obstacles such as lack of transportation and Canada's winter climate further impede the attainment of financial security.

Studies of rural people's attitudes and beliefs (Farley 1982) point to an inherently traditional, conservative bias. It is a historical tradition in agrarian societies that wives and children are legally under the direction, protection, and control of the landowner. Any wife or child who attempted to escape from this rule was ordered back to the master. Modern rural societies have mellowed somewhat, but the legacy remains. Wives and children are often financially dependent; the rural church provides ideological support to old traditions by preaching the virtues of the dependent status of women; and community services are practically nonexistent (Collier 1984). The conservatism of rural attitudes often makes it difficult for a woman to seek and hold employment, particularly in nontraditional, higher-paying jobs. This leaves many women underemployed, if not unemployed, and financially dependent.

Rural women have also been chronically excluded and underrepresented at all levels of decision making (Canadian Rural Development Council 1979; Research, Action, Education Center 1982). When rural women were surveyed, only 8 per cent of the women felt they had parity with men in community decision making (Potter and Dustan 1983).

This lack of decision-making power in the community is evident despite the high degree of community involvement of rural women (Cooper 1979). Britton (1984) reports on a study of farm women in Prince Edward Island done by Leona McIsaac. McIsaac found that the average woman put in 10.5 hours per month in community work and held membership in two groups. Communities and families place high expectations on rural women. Many small communities offer a large number of associations, equal to those available in larger centers, but the volunteer workers who develop these groups are few in numbers so the burden is heavier for each individual (Manitoba Advisory Council on the Status of Women 1984).

Rural women's political invisibility parallels the lack of political power among women in general. Women are neither socialized for political competition nor encouraged to participate in political activities. We lack political role models and the opportunities to develop the necessary leadership skills. Consequently, we are less confident of our political capabilities (Bokemeir and Tait 1980). This lack of political efficacy must be considered in light of the fact that women only gained suffrage seventy years ago (1917, both federally and in Manitoba), after a campaign that took slightly more than half a century (Brodie and Vickers 1982).

Rural women have a higher degree of political invisibility than their urban sisters, but we can find hope in rural women's longstanding commitment to community involvement and their emerging sensitivity and willingness to be involved in more political action on their own behalf. Remember, rural Manitoban women already have at least one role model; Nellie McClung was a rural woman.

The personal power of women, or lack of it, can be understood as a political issue. The limiting of economic and political power is directly connected to the lessening of personal power in the cycle of oppression.

Haussman and Halseth (1983) found that depression is a problem of epidemic proportions for rural women. They link depression to low income, lack of social and educational opportunities, inadequate child care resources, transportation difficulties, the demands of a traditional family role regardless of a woman's employment, and isolation. Evans and Cooperstock (1983) confirm this analysis in their study of the psychosocial problems facing rural women in primary resource communities such as Thompson or Fort McMurray. Women in primary resource communities face more severe isolation from other communities and from extended family, which is compounded by a high turnover of friends. Evans and Cooperstock cite evidence regarding the exceptionally high rates of prescribing minor tranquilizers and anti-depressants to women, a problem also noted in Ireland's (1983) study of farm women. Isolation is of primary importance, with the following factors contributing: difficult climate; poor or nonexistent public transportation within the community; lack of child care facilities; lack of appropriate public places to meet other women during the day or evening; and the emotional isolation of living in a male-oriented culture.

While urban and rural women alike suffer from symptoms of oppression, the geographic isolation of rural women directly affects the availability of services. Appropriate mental health services for rural women are sadly lacking. Delivery of services within the rural community is generally more expensive than in urban areas, both because of the lower socioeconomic status of rural communities – meaning less local contribution to federal and provincial services – and because fewer clients are concentrated in a given space, meaning that fixed-service locations are less feasible (Farley et al. 1982; Collier 1984).

The existence of fewer services, combined with a more traditional view of women's roles, leaves women who are in need of mental health services without them. When services are present, they are often only available on an itinerant basis, delivered by statutory-type social service agencies.

Rural women often must seek help from agencies that view women as mentally unhealthy (Broverman, Clarkson, and Frank 1970), that do not consider the social context of her difficulties (Weissman 1971; Penfold, and Walker 1983), and whose therapeutic goal has been to move women toward a greater acceptance of their presumed inferior status (Russel 1979). Helen Levine (1982, 77) presents an excellent summary of the deficits of traditional systems in helping women gain empowerment:

By and large, women have found [that] helpers stress adjustment rather than change; individual, not collective or political solutions; personal pathology; weakness rather than strength; the psyche unrelated to economic

and social hazards in women's lives; and the authority of male experts, male
management and male decision-makers in and beyond the home ... the goal
of ensuring that women remain in their place, serving others and sacrificing
their own separate, adult, human rights has often been found lurking un-
derneath the subtle and sophisticated surface of therapy, counselling and
treatment.

Rural women need nontraditional services to begin to heal the
pain of invisibility and isolation. Since those in control of the economic and political power are slow to acknowledge the gaps in services or to provide funding to develop the services required, rural
women are finding ways to examine their lives and work towards
empowering themselves. This is happening throughout rural and
northern Manitoba through support and action groups. The remainder of this article will focus on the value of these groups – all-
women groups in the self-help tradition (Hill 1984; Women's Counselling, Referral and Education Center 1984) – as one way to begin
to deal with some of the stress inherent in the lives of rural women.

Women exist as an oppressed group with one major characteristic
(other than their majority in numbers) which sets them apart from
other oppressed groups. Women live side by side with the oppressor.
Women and men are bound together in a socially sanctioned sex-
gender system through sexuality, marriage, and procreation. Many
women, particularly those who live with men, are segregated from
other non-kin women and are prevented from recognizing the
sources of their powerlessness, a recognition other groups have
learned in the ghetto (Lipman-Blumen 1984). This segregation,
heightened by rural factors related to isolation, results in few opportunities for women to share their common plight, to validate each
other, and to free ideas and anger to work on their own behalf.
Here "own" is the operative word, as women have long been organized to work on behalf of others (Mackie 1983).

Studies in speech habits (Kramer, Thorne, and Henley 1978) have
shown that the patterns between men and women resemble those
between other dominants and subordinates. Men talk more, take
more turns at talking, initiate 96 per cent of all interruptions, and
in that way control the topic of conversation. When women interrupt
to regain the floor they are ignored. Apart from men, women are
more free to speak, to develop relationships with each other, and to
acknowledge strengths in themselves (Carlock and Martin 1977). In
fact, one of the most positive outcomes of women's groups is the
rediscovery of the pleasures and fulfillment of interpersonal relations with other women (Walker 1981). A strong network of women

friends is crucial in helping women to enjoy life fully and to reduce dependency on men (Caplan 1981).

A primary characteristic of women's groups is the emphasis they place on the social and political factors which relate to women's individual situations. Given the way women have been socialized, and given our present status and roles in society, the unveiling of the sociopolitical context helps women to recognize that social changes are necessary for significant improvement to occur in our lives. This enables women to begin to differentiate between what they can individually control and what requires political action. This process sometimes involves a major alteration in women's attitudes towards, and understanding of, the world and of women's ability to enact change. Cherniss (1972) found that after only a few months in a consciousness raising group, women seemed to undergo a number of changes in attitudes and behaviour, moving towards the direction of independence, autonomy, activity, mobility, self-esteem and self-acceptance.

All-women groups provide a validation of women's life experience as we feel it, as we react to it. According to Levine (1982), this validation is a significant experience for most women because it implies respect, dignity, and trust, rare commodities in a patriarchial system. Rural women, strongly affected by the overwhelmingly conservative, male-dominated milieu in which they live, are often convinced that they are "a little crazy" if they do not accept the status quo. "What is wrong with me, if I am not happy being Mrs John Doe?"

In groups, things that have been thought of as personal peculiarities begin to look amazingly like women's collective psyche. This awareness begins the healing process. Nadeau (1982), discussing mutual aid in resource-based communities, stated that the success and appeal of these groups is largely due to the contact and support they offer to women experiencing considerable physical and emotional isolation.

The attainment of personal goals for individual women and political goals for women collectively are not separate. Often the personal experience of accepting the reality of women's oppression stirs a need to do something, no matter how small, to alter our lives, our community, or both (Women's Self Help Network 1984). The activity of lobbying for social change can provide the focal point to bring together women for personal support. It is this author's contention that the integration of self-care and political involvement is critical. Interviews with five women's groups across rural Manitoba substantiate this belief (Graveline 1985).

Support, often described as "connection to like-minded women," was considered essential for all of the groups. Other priorities included: personal and public education on themes such as pornography, media monitoring, violence against women, and abortion; outreach or connection with other women and women's groups on issues of mutual concern; political action, from an individual woman approaching a local merchant about the pornography on his shelves to lobbying the premier on the needs of rural women; and the provision of services to women, such as safe houses for battered women or referrals to nontraditional professionals.

The size of the group affects its function, with larger groups being more productive for political functions and smaller groups providing better individual involvement (Home 1981). Function may also affect size. More women may be more attracted to groups which offer sociopolitical solutions to the challenges of rural life than to those that emphasize the more traditional foci of individual problem-solving or community support. Regardless of stated function or size, the groups interviewed were all involved in the often complicated juggling that goes on to balance personal support for members with activity and action on behalf of others.

In summary, rural women have been ignored as a group in need of special consideration. They have been made invisible economically, politically, and personally. The factors contributing to their invisibility include fewer employment and training opportunities; time constraints; lack of services; conservative attitudes and beliefs; and geographic and emotional isolation. These factors, when combined with the sexism inherent in our socialization, social structures, and traditional helping systems, produce a group of women with many needs and with little access to resources with which to meet those needs. The structure of women's support and action groups, using feminist strategies designed to enhance power in women's lives, serves to begin the process of including women in personal and political decision making. Increased knowledge, provided through discussion and analysis of the issue and transmitted to the community through public education and political action, begins to alter the power structure. The inclusion of women combats invisibility and isolation, the greatest foes of rural women.

Our society has spent much time and energy in fashioning chains to restrain women from collectively and individually claiming their fair share of economic, political, and personal power. Bringing rural women together, to end our isolation and to join our urban sisters, can only result in strengthening our voice and in eventually breaking down historical traditions. Women will reclaim their rights; support and action groups are one way to begin the process of empowerment. We face many barriers, but there is joy in the struggle.

REFERENCES

Armstrong, P. and H. Armstrong 1982. *The Double Ghetto.* Toronto: Mc-Clelland and Stewart.

Bokemeir, J. and J. Tait 1980. "Women as Power Actors: A Comparative Study of Rural Communities." *Rural Sociology* 45: 238–55.

Britton, H. 1984. "Farm Women's Roles Seldom Examined." *Manitoba Cooperative*, 29 August 1984 issue.

Broverman, I., *et al.* 1970. "Sex Role Stereotypes and Clinical Judgements of Mental Health." *Journal of Consulting and Clinical Psychology* 34: 1–7.

Brodie, J. and J. Vickers 1982. *Canadian Women in Politics: An Overview.* Ottawa: Canadian Research Institute for the Advancement of Women.

Caplan, P. 1981. *Between Women: Lowering the Barriers.* Toronto: Personal Library.

Carlock, C.J. and Martin 1977. "Sex Composition and the Intensive Group Experience." *Social Work* 22: 27–32.

Cherniss, C. 1972. "Personality and Ideology: A Personological Study of Women's Liberation." *Psychiatry* 35: 109–25.

Clark, S. and A.S. Harvey 1976. "The Sexual Division of Labour: The Use of Time." *Atlantis* 1: 46–66.

Cooper, P. 1979. "Women as Advocates in Their Communities." *Atlantis* 4: 121–8.

Council on Rural Development Canada 1979. "Rural Women's Study: Their Work, Their Needs, and Their Role in Rural Development." Unpublished ms. on file.

Eichler, M. 1983. *Families in Canada Today.* Toronto: Gage.

Evans, J. and R. Cooperstock 1983. "Psycho-social Problems of Women in Primary Resource Communities." *Canadian Journal of Community Mental Health* 1: 59–66.

Farley, O. W. *et al.* 1982. *Rural Social Work Practice.* New York: The Free Press.

Fitzgerald, M., M. Wolfe, and C. Guberman, eds. 1982. *Still Ain't Satisfied.* Toronto: The Women's Press.

Graveline, M.J. 1985. *Support Groups for Rural Women: Decreasing Invisibility and Isolation.* MSW thesis, University of Manitoba.

Haussman, M. and J. Halseth 1983. "Re-examining Women's Roles: A Feminist Approach to Decreasing Depression in Women." *Social Work With Groups* Fall/Winter, 105–15.

Smith, D. and S. David 1975. *Women Look at Psychiatry*. Vancouver: Press Gang.

Turner, J. and L. Emery 1983. *Perspectives on Women in the 1980s*. Winnipeg: University of Manitoba Press.

Walker, L. 1981. "Are Women's Groups Different?" *Psychotherapy Theory, Research and Practice* 18: 240–5.

Weisstein, N. 1971. "Psychology Constructs the Female." In V. Gornich and B. Moran, eds., *Women in Sexist Society*. New York: Basic Books.

Women's Self Help Network 1984. *Working Together For a Change*. Campbell River, B.C.: Ptarmigan Press.

Hill, K. 1984. *Helping You Helps Me: A Guidebook for Self-help Groups*. Ottawa: Canadian Council on Social Development.

Home, A. 1981. "A Study of Change in Women's Consciousness-raising Groups." *Canadian Journal of Social Work Education* 6: 1–24.

Ireland, G. 1983. *The Farmer Takes a Wife*. Chelsey: Concerned Farm Women.

Kramer, C., B. Thorne, and N. Henley "Review Essay: Language and Communication." *Signs* 3: 638–51.

Levine, H. 1982. "The Personal Is Political: Feminism and the Helping Professions." In A. Miles and G. Finn, eds., *Feminism in Canada: From Pressure to Politics*. Montreal: Black Rose Books.

Lipman-Blumen, J. 1984. *Gender Roles and Power*. Englewood, New Jersey: Prentice-Hall.

Mackie, M. 1983. *Exploring Gender Relations: A Canadian Perspective*. Toronto: Butterworths.

Manitoba Advisory Council on the Status of Women 1984. "Some Concerns of Rural Women." Manuscript on file.

McGhee, M. 1984. *Women in Rural Life*. Toronto: Ministry of Agriculture and Food.

Meissner, M. and P. Humphreys 1975. "No Exit for Wives: Sexual Division of Labour and the Cumulation of Housework Demands." *Canadian Review of Sociology and Anthropology* 12: 424–33.

Nadeau, D. 1982. "Women and Self-help in Resource-based Communities." *Resources for Feminist Research* 11: 65–66.

National Council on Welfare 1979. *Women and Poverty*. Ottawa.

Norman, E. and A. Mancuso 1980. *Women's Issues and Social Work Practice*. Ithaca, N.Y.: F.E. Peacock.

O'Connell, D. 1983. "Poverty: A Feminine Complaint." In J. Turner and L. Emery, eds., *Perspectives On Women in the 1980s*. Winnipeg: University of Manitoba Press.

Penefold, S. and G. Walker 1983. *Women and the Psychiatric Paradox*. Montreal: Eden Press.

Potter, C. and L. Dustan 1983. "Data Analysis with Respect to a Survey of Members of the Manitoba Action Committee on the Status of Women and Other Women in Areas Outside of Brandon and Winnipeg." Manuscript on file, Manitoba Action Committee on the Status of Women, Brandon, Manitoba.

Research, Action, and Education Center 1982. "Keeping Women Down on the Farm." *Resources for Feminist Research* 11: 13–4.

Russel, M. 1979. "Feminist Therapy: A Critical Examination." *The Social Worker* Summer/Fall: 61–5.

Saskatchewan Labour 1981. "Never Just a Wife." *About Women*, January/ February.

Women, Knowledge, and Well-Being
Les femmes, la connaissance, et le mieux-être

CLAIRE V. DE LA DURANTAYE

La plénitude, du mythe à la divagation

La plénitude sera présentée ici comme un concept décrivant une série d'attitudes, de perceptions et de formes d'appréhension du réel que retrace une analyse de divers discours de femmes, particulièrement ceux qui entourent la façon dont les femmes abordent la connaissance, le savoir. Elle sera définie comme cette recherche d'une *globalité* dans tout instant, dans toute réalité, dans tous les objets et les êtres. Nous tenterons de démontrer le double potentiel révolutionnaire de ce concept pour les femmes et pour la pensée féministe. C'est-à-dire, d'une part, de poser le concept de plénitude comme *caractéristique épistémologique fondamentale* de l'acte de connaître des femmes, cette caractéristique de la pensée des femmes se révélant essentielle au développement d'une pensée féministe originale (nonrépétitive) et indispensable à la construction d'une nouvelle épistémologie (Irigaray 1987). D'autre part, le concept de plénitude se pose comme *fondement politique* de la situation sociale des femmes. Cette manière de savoir, cette manière de se sentir et de voir des femmes opposeraient celles-ci aux projets finalistes et technicistes des hommes (obligeant ceux-ci à la domination de celles-là). Une nouvelle dimension de l'exploitation des femmes émerge ainsi de la lutte entre la globalité féminine et le finalisme masculin. Nous terminerons par une relecture des principales contradictions sociales actuelles à la lumière de cette nouvelle dualité.

Well-Being: From Myth to Holism

Well-being is presented here as a concept which describes a series of attitudes, perceptions, and ways of apprehending reality that can be traced through an analysis of various female discourses, specifically those which underpin the female approach to cognizance and to various forms of knowledge. Well-being is defined as the search for *universality* at every instant, within every reality, in all objects and persons. I attempt to demonstrate the revolutionary potential of this concept both for women and for feminist thought. In other words, I am proposing, on the one hand, the concept of well-being as the basic epistemological characteristic of women's approach to knowledge. This characteristic of female thought is fundamental to the development of an original and nonrepetitive feminist thought and indispensable to the development of a new epistemology (Irigaray 1987). On the other hand, the concept of well-being may be seen as the basis for any political project designed to modify the female social situation. This holistic approach of knowing, seeing, and being aware of society and of themselves places women in diametric opposition to the divisive, reductionist, technical male approach and forces them into domination by men). Understanding well-being in this way provides a new dimension to the exploitation of women, allowing it to be seen as a result of the struggle between female universality and male determinism. I finish by reviewing major current social contradictions in the light of this new duality.

INTRODUCTION

On a longtemps dit que les femmes étaient passives. Simplement c'est qu'elles recherchent quelque chose que les hommes, eux, ne recherchent pas. En rassemblant des témoignages divers de femmes dont les pensées ou les oeuvres ont marqué, un concept émerge qui circonscrit bien cette vision particulière qu'ont les femmes des êtres et des choses. Ce concept, c'est celui de la plénitude. Ce que nous proposons ici constitue un essai de définition de ce qu'est la plénitude, de l'importance et de la portée qu'a, à nos yeux, ce concept. Nous présentons la plénitude comme un attribut essentiellement féminin, décrivant une série d'attitudes, de perceptions et de formes d'appréhension du réel que les femmes adoptent pour parler d'elles, de leurs aspirations et de la société dans son devenir. Nous la définissons comme cette vision d'unité absolue des êtres et des choses, comme une fusion de tous les instants et de tous les espaces (abstraits comme concrets), où toutes les réalités se retrouvent sans qu'aucune ne disparaisse dans cette fusion, au profit d'une autre. La plénitude, chez les femmes, c'est la recherche du plein en opposition à la recherche, chez les hommes, de la finalité c'est-à-dire des fins, des limites.

Un tel concept de plénitude est particulièrement important pour qui veut comprendre les rapports de sexes dans nos sociétés. Celles-ci, en effet, souffrent d'une manière aiguë des conséquences de la domination masculine instaurée sur toute chose. Ce concept permet, d'une part, de saisir davantage la différence féminine et de guider l'action concrète des femmes aujourd'hui. Mais, croyons-nous d'autre part, il peut également fonder une sorte de « révolution paradigmatique » des connaissances (Kuhn 1983, 283). La plénitude pourrait en effet être ce concept fondamental favorisant l'établissement d'une nouvelle science et d'une nouvelle éthique en se substituant aux objectifs traditionnels de la science, qui sont: la découverte des finalités dites « objectives » des êtres et des choses, la recherche de la « globalité », etc.

L'attitude de l'homme de science n'est nullement celle d'un propriétaire terrien ... au contraire, lorsqu'un nouveau terrain lui échoit, il se précipite à ses frontières et n'est plus obsédé que par une question: que cachent les murs qui le bornent ... » (Jacquard 1982, 13).

La plénitude offrirait de nouvelles avenues épistémologiques aux sciences: l'harmonie des parties, l'union du micro et du macrocosme, de l'espace et du temps.

Les femmes correspondent au singulier universel. En elles, elles allient le plus singulier et le plus universel. Leur identité se tient dans la nonscission systématique de la nature et de l'esprit, dans la retouche de ces deux universels. La femme est entière et universelle, universelle si entière. Notre culture a là aussi inversé l'ordre des choses (Irigaray 1987, 126).

Nos réflexions seront donc groupées sous trois rubriques dans un style plutôt schématique, compte tenu du temps qui nous est imparti. Le premier groupe de réflexions portera sur le sens du mot plénitude. La question que l'on pose est: existe-t-il un sentiment de plénitude? Une définition du terme et du concept est-elle possible? Le deuxième groupe de réflexions portera sur la valeur stratégique de ce concept comme réponse possible aux contradictions de la société actuelle. La question posée sera: la plénitude, cette recherche de plénitude, existe-t-elle encore aujourd'hui? Doit-on la mettre en valeur dans notre engagement social et politique, nous les femmes? Et finalement, le troisième groupe de réflexions tentera de donner quelques éléments de propositions pour un nouveau paradigme qu'inspirerait ce concept de plénitude et qui permettrait enfin l'accès des femmes au statut de sujet de connaissance (Marcil-Lacoste 1983). Nous conclurons cet exposé en proposant l'adoption de la plénitude comme dimension réelle et théorique des femmes; comme concept universel. Nous souhaitons voir se poursuivre la recherche et

l'approfondissement de ce concept qui fonde, selon nous, la différence des femmes dans notre monde.

LA PLÉNITUDE : MYTHE OU DIVAGATION ?

> Pauvre et romantique, elle refait le monde de
> choses magnifiques. Aimer pour aimer. (Chanson populaire)

Le mythe consiste en une représentation du monde que se donne
l'esprit humain pour comprendre et unifier les perceptions qu'il tire
de la réalité de son environnement. La fonction première du mythe
est « d'aider les êtres humains à supporter l'angoisse et l'absurdité
de leur condition » (Jacob 1981, 29). Le mythe ne constitue pas une
connaissance scientifique de la réalité. Il tient davantage à l'imagination et aux désirs qu'à la réalité constatée. Cependant, la constance
d'un mythe à travers l'histoire tend à signifier des valeurs et croyances
des hommes et des femmes que la science n'explique pas encore ou
réfute, mais que ceux-ci et celles-ci maintiennent dans une culture,
c'est-à-dire une certaine pertinence sociale.

La divagation. « Divaguer, du bas latin: divagaris, signifie errer ça et là;
penser sans sujet précis, ne pas raisonner correctement, parler d'une manière absurde ... » (Thomas 1979, 7).

Depuis trente ans, l'épanouissement féminin, cette dimension féminine au bonheur, avait quelque peu été oublié, voire rejeté. Il
nous paraissait qu'il avait, dans le meilleur des cas, été confondu
avec le mythe de la femme amante, avec l'amour. Confondu avec la
manière dont on souhaitait que les femmes aiment. Dans le pire des
cas, il représentait l'image même de la domination masculine sur la
femme: une image de la femme passive et asservie.

   Il nous est donc apparu intéressant de profiter de ce colloque pour
tenter de creuser davantage ce mythe (?) ou cette divagation (?) de
la plénitude chez la femme; d'une idée de bonheur propre à elle.
La femme serait-elle cette essence mystérieuse, différente de
l'homme, ce don total, qui se livrerait tout entière à lui par Amour?
(S'y consumant sans laisser de trace!) Ou bien, cette forme d'amour
est-il totalement et entièrement créé par une culture masculine?
Sommes-nous toutes de ces femmes qui aiment trop (Norwood 1986,
304)? Ou encore, cette importance de l'amour dans nos vies, cette
manière d'être constamment liées aux autres, ne représente-t-elle
pas *aussi* une forme *d'être* particulière aux femmes? Comme une
manière d'exister et de rechercher sa substance vive? Si oui, cet

amour des femmes envers elles et les autres pourrait être une manifestation d'un besoin de plénitude cherchant à s'exprimer dans
cette société masculine.

Mais ce qu'on nomme à tort « romantique » provient en réalité de ce qui,
en nous, est parfaitement indestructible, robuste, originel: de notre force
vitale même, qui seule peut affronter le monde extérieur, car elle a la
certitude que l'intérieur et l'extérieur ont les même racines » (Andreas,
Salome 1977, 26).

   Quelques témoignages. L. Bernier et I. Perreault, deux artistes,
considèrent que leurs oeuvres, leur art, sont l'expression d'un moment d'union, de communion entre des réalités qui s'opposent, mais
auxquelles elles ne peuvent renoncer.[1] C'est le besoin du tout pour
se réaliser. Ces mêmes sentiments de plein, d'indissociabilité,
d'amour se retrouvent également chez des auteures telles Lou
Andréas Salomé,[2] Camille Claudel,[3] et pourquoi pas la célèbre ab-
besse Héloïse.[4] Ces femmes cherchent à se définir par un besoin de
plénitude, un sentiment d'amour qui embrasse toute leur intériorité
et leur être.
   Nous pouvons également inverser la perspective. C'est-à-dire recueillir des témoignages où il est dit que l'incapacité des femmes à
atteindre cette plénitude provoque une cassure psychologique chez
elles, un isolement, un *vide*. Ces femmes qui aiment trop, ne luttent-
elles pas pour combler un vide immanent (Norwood 1986)? Julia
Kristeva (1987), psychiatre, explique dans son dernier livre (*Soleil
Noir*) le phénomène dépressif chez les femmes comme l'expression
irréparable d'un *vide*, d'une *absence*. Marilyn French (1980) dans *Les
bons sentiments* parle du besoin qu'ont les femmes de toujours vouloir
recoller les morceaux de leurs réalités éparses. Citons à nouveau
Luce Irigaray (1987, 74):

Si les femmes manquent de Dieu, elles ne peuvent communiquer ni com-
munier entre elles. Il faut, il leur faut, l'infini pour partager un peu. Sinon,
le partage entraîne fusion-confusion, division et déchirements en elle(s),
entre elles. Si je ne me rapporte pas à quelqu'horizon d'accomplissement
de mon genre, je ne peux partager en protégeant mon devenir.

Également l'opinion des hommes, des *autres* sur cette attitude et ce
besoin profond de plénitude ressenti par les femmes. Leur témoi-
gnage constitue un aspect révélateur intéressant de ce sentiment et
du fondement de son existence. Par exemple, ne rapporte-t-on pas
que Freud aurait écrit, en parlant de Lou Andréas Salomé, la phrase

suivante: « je sépare l'un l'autre et vous réunissez ce qui a été séparé en une unité supérieure » (Andreas Salomé 1977, xiv). Elle se sentait, elle-même, comme une « image symbolique » permettant aux autres (comprendre, ici, aux hommes) de mettre « en branle l'association amour-savoir-désir, dont la femme est le support » (xv). Rodin, au sommet de sa gloire, usa de toute son influence pour bloquer l'achat par l'État français d'une oeuvre de Camille Claudel. Commande qui aurait permis à cette dernière de résoudre ses difficultés financières. Il le fit pour empêcher « que sa vie intime ne soit exposée sur la place publique » (Cassar 1988, 370). Laissant ainsi la géniale sculpteure sombrer dans la déchéance *sociale*, puis subir l'enfermement.

Ce qui frappe, ici, c'est l'existence chez les femmes du sentiment du tout. La plénitude existe. Elle n'est pas un mythe, ni une divagation. Cependant exprimée socialement, cette force serait source de bien des difficultés. Reproche de trop de passion, d'excès de sentiments, etc. Ce *trop* chez les femmes leur vaudrait, lorsqu'elles essaieraient de s'exprimer socialement, d'être considérées comme inadaptées. C'est le mythe de la faible femme, du « sexe faible. »

D'autre part, lorsque la société masculine parviendrait à canaliser à ses propres fins ce sentiment, à le « privatiser », la plénitude des femmes deviendrait alors cause de troubles pour les femmes, mais source de dynamisme chez les hommes. C'est le mythe de la femme passive. La société masculine aurait ainsi créé des mythes pour s'approprier ce sentiment de plénitude chez les femmes.

La plénitude n'est pas un mythe ni une divagation. Elle désigne un rapport très précis des femmes à l'univers. Elle caractérise leur manière d'être et de faire puisque, chez les femmes, les deux ne se dissocient pas. C'est la négation de la plénitude qui est un mythe.

LA VALEUR STRATÉGIQUE DU CONCEPT DE PLÉNITUDE

L'histoire et en particulier l'histoire des femmes est significative de ce point de vue. La disparition progressive des femmes du système social d'organisation et de représentation, leur domination sociale par les hommes marquent, selon plusieurs auteures (Irigaray 1987; Lindsey et Duffim 1985, 212), la fin de l'harmonie des hommes et des femmes en communauté, avec leur environnement, avec l'univers. Cet abandon signifie la perte d'une complémentarité des devenirs, d'une plénitude des êtres et des choses. Elle est remplacée par une objectivation, un partitionnement des différentes composantes de ce même univers: le corps, la nature, la psychologie, la raison, etc. que les hommes se plaisent à contrôler, manipuler et diriger selon leurs désirs.

Or, la plénitude, si elle fut vécue sous une société matriarcale (ou du moins plus égalitaire) (Irigaray 1987), devient dans le contexte actuel une quête urgente et vitale à la survie des femmes. Le finalisme masculin généralisant et neutralisant toutes les essences qui lui sont étrangères retranche en effet de plus en plus les réalités des femmes vers le non-dit, vers la négation jusqu'à une absorption et une disparition complète du féminin. La plénitude serait, pour nous, le véritable enjeu du mouvement féministe actuel: réaffirmer notre perspective de différentiation et de fusion comme indispensable à la construction d'un monde viable et heureux.

L'occident qui a inventé l'amour n'a pas atteint la pensée de l'amour. ... L'espèce humaine entière s'efforce millénairement de dissocier la fécondation et la volupté. Ce qui a permis la séparation fictive et réelle à la fois du corps et de l'esprit » (Lefebvre 1985, 114).

Il nous apparaît donc que nous vivons dans cette société une « lutte » à finir (?) entre deux projets de l'universel desquels découlent toutes nos conditions de vie et d'existence. Le premier de ces projets, dominant et en voie de réalisation totale, concerne cette société hiérarchique, au masculin, imposant le finalisme technologique et la compartimentation des êtres et des choses sous contrôle du Père. Un système où se côtoient les hasards et le téléologique. De l'autre, le projet du devenir multiple, du dépassement et de la substance sous le signe de la femme féconde, pourvoyeuse comme la nature et, harmonisante avec ce qui l'entoure. Projet refoulé aujourd'hui au rang du mythe par la société post-moderne mais qui contient, là, le germe du seul projet de société vraiment original que puissent apporter les femmes. Approcherions-nous du moment où nous, les femmes, perdrons complètement toute trace de ce que nous avons été et, par conséquent de ce que nous voulons être?

Pourquoi disons-nous que cette société post-moderne est masculine? Tout d'abord, parce qu'elle a été faite par des hommes. Ceci est historiquement vérifiable. Puis, parce qu'elle exclut d'une façon systématique les femmes. Ceci est statistiquement vérifiable. Et en troisième lieu, parce que sa logique de développement correspond en tous points à celle des hommes: une abstraction excessive, une volonté de domination pour amener à des fins prédéterminées, un besoin de diviser, etc.

Ce type d'explication, de fonctionnement, me semble correspondre au modèle de sexualité – masculine – décrit par Freud: tension, décharge, retour
à l'hosméostasie, etc. (Irigaray 1987, 90).

Voilà pourquoi il nous faut étudier un peu plus précisément ce
qu'est cette société post-moderne, ses fondements et ses contradictions. Et ce, afin d'y découvrir ce que la plénitude peut apporter
comme stratégie de changement.

Tout d'abord les fondements de la société actuelle (de la Durantaye
1988, 90). La société post-moderne repose sur trois forces principales: la science et la technologie, l'organisation et les idéologies
(Lyotard 1979, 112). Ces forces ne sont pas nécessairement récentes,
comme celle de la technologie par exemple. Mais les transformations
récentes qu'elles ont subies, la généralisation de leur application à
tous les rapports sociaux (travail, vie familiale, vie sociale, rapports
hommes-femmes, etc.) en font les véhicules principaux des conditions et du mode de vie de chacun et chacune de nous. Ces forces
ont une action destructrice sur le social. Leur action combinée détruit
progressivement le tissu social, les liens entre ses différentes composantes. Ce sont les impératifs de la rentabilité et du profit, de la
« rationalité objective » du progrès scientifique et du contrôle social
qui constituent le moteur de ces forces. Ils servent à la réalisation
de son projet (Meister 1975, 312).

Cette société engendre ses propres contradictions. Nous voudrions
en donner trois qui nous paraissent particulièrement importantes.
La première est la généralisation du culte de l'objet entretenu par
ce système. Les femmes, depuis longtemps vouées au rôle d'objet
(sexuel, de consommation, etc.) voient maintenant se joindre à elles
un nombre grandissant de groupes sociaux (« le bel âge », « la femme
de *carrière* », « l'entrepreneure », etc.). Ces groupes, ramenés au rôle
de figurants, ont perdu toute identité propre et toute capacité d'agir
sur leur destin. Il doivent s'en remettre aux desseins, aux projets de
ceux qui détiennent le pouvoir. Plus précisément, ils doivent chercher à s'identifier aux modèles des fonctions sociales auxquelles ils
prétendent. Il y a donc multiplication des objets avec « risque » d'interaction entre eux (Bertrand 1987, 322)!

En second lieu, il y a la confusion actuelle entre sphère privée et
sphère publique. La société masculine se décrète d'ordre public. Elle
se dit universelle. C'est d'ailleurs elle qui a imposé cette coupure
politique privé/publique. C'est elle, en effet, qui contrôle les différents rapports sociaux de travail, loisir, de production-reproduction.
Dans un tel contexte, les femmes sont réduites à un rôle sexuel et
de maternage, c'est-à-dire à un rôle privé. Or, au fur et à mesure

que l'organisation du système masculin se complexifie et s'étend à l'ensemble des rapports sociaux, une nécessité s'impose: celle d'étendre la coupure privée/publique à d'autres types d'organisations et fonctions sociales. C'est l'éclatement de la sphère « privée » réservée jusqu'ici aux femmes. C'est la coupure sexe/genre qui apparaît.

En troisième et dernier lieu, c'est la contradiction issue de la lutte pour la production/reproduction sociale. La société masculine s'est érigée sur la base du principe de l'organisation et du contrôle social afin de s'approprier la capacité reproductive biologique, mais aussi sociale des femmes. Pour enlever à la société (hommes-femmes) dans son ensemble, la capacité de devenir *ensemble*. Ce refus de l'altérité entre hommes et femmes entraîne la disparition des femmes. Celles-ci sont femmes et mères. Supprimer un terme supprime l'essence. Cela supprime également la différence, la capacité de changer, d'innover et de se développer. L'homme en tuant la femme, tuerait donc son propre avenir (Irigaray 1987).

La plénitude s'oppose comme vision du monde au projet de la société post-moderne. À la tendance à diviser, contrôler, abstraire et plier à ses propres fins l'ensemble de l'univers, elle oppose l'harmonie, l'union, le respect des différences, la création par le dépassement des entités, la fusion. La plénitude unit, renforce, vit l'intensité de soi et de l'autre, elle est ouverte. Sa logique en est une de respect de chacune des entités. Pour elle, le domaine du sensible (concret) est en parfaite harmonie avec celui de la pensée. L'un ne peut exister sans l'autre. Elle ne tend pas vers une connaissance spécialisée, mais vers une connaissance pleine des êtres et des choses. Comme un nouvel humanisme. Oui, le concept de plénitude est révolutionnaire, car il dépasse et transforme la logique dichotomique du système social masculin actuel.

Voyons maintenant, rapidement, comment il peut transformer la connaissance, les fondements de cet acte de connaître.

VERS UN NOUVEAU PARADIGME

Dans l'introduction à cet exposé nous parlions du potentiel du concept de plénitude dans l'établissement d'un nouveau paradigme. Nous allons maintenant donner quelques jalons de réflexions à ce raisonnement.

Le concept de plénitude, que nous avons attribué aux femmes seulement, est issu du rapport mère-fille. Il touche à des valeurs d'ordre universel. C'est-à-dire que, d'abord et avant toute chose, une femme ne perçoit pas l'univers, la vie, la mort, la connaissance, etc.

comme l'homme (Irigaray 1987). Tout devenir, toute connaissance de notre devenir est *sexué*. Nous, les femmes, il se réalise par la quête de la plénitude.

Pour devenir, il est nécessaire d'avoir un genre ou une essence (dès lors sexuée) comme horizon. Sinon, le devenir reste partiel et assujetti. Devenir parties ou multiples sans futur propre aboutit à s'en remettre à l'autre ou l'autre de l'autre pour son rassemblement » (Irigaray 1987, 73).

Ces valeurs d'ordre universel sont donc inévitablement sexuées. Elles transpireront et détermineront la connaissance dont, forcément, autant la culture, qui est une connaissance concrète, que la science qui est une connaissance abstraite du monde. Or, si toute connaissance est ainsi sexuée dès le départ, celle, actuelle, est *masculine*. Justement parce que les femmes, les valeurs des femmes, les connaissances des femmes en ont été exclues (Harding 1983). Cette exclusion s'est faite sous l'égide d'un certain rationalisme fondé sur l'abstraction – neutralisation (Lefebvre 1979, 292).

Comme le fait Luce Irigaray elle-même (Irigaray 1984, 200), nous fondons cette masculinisation des connaissances sur la nécessité vitale que ressent l'homme de contrôler son rapport à la nature, son rapport à la société. L'homme serait plus agressif, dominant, car marqué par sa différence d'avec sa mère, sa séparation de celle-ci. Le paradigme scientifique masculin répondrait à ces valeurs.

Le paradigme féminin propose une reprise en main par les femmes et les hommes (unies) de leur devenir. Les femmes sont les forces qui unissent. Ne sont-elles pas « entre »? En affirmant la valeur de la plénitude, les femmes éclaireraient le sens et la démarche de la science. Elles permettraient ainsi une recentration de l'humanité sur elle-même, sur son bonheur. Ce que l'homme recherche, finalement, c'est la femme. Pourquoi ne l'admet-il pas tout simplement?

CONCLUSION

Ce qui frappe lorsque nous entrons au musée d'Orsay à Paris c'est la surreprésentation des artistes masculins d'une part et d'autre part, la surreprésentation des formes féminines. En fait, on distingue mal la femme de toutes ces formes arrondies de l'art, du meuble et de la sculpture. L'art c'est l'harmonie, les liens, les passages, d'une réalité à une autre toutes présentes, entières dans cet espèce d'effacement vis-à-vis de l'autre. Et ainsi voit-on la femme: toute présente en permettant ce passage de l'homme à l'homme, de l'homme à l'univers. Sa plénitude à ce moment-ci, c'est sa discrétion, ses formes arrondies...

La plénitude n'est pas un mythe. Elle n'est pas une divagation non plus. Elle existe. Les femmes en souffrent (souvent) ou en jouissent (plus rarement). Les hommes en profitent. Les femmes sont la plénitude des hommes. Mais cette attitude fondamentale des femmes à être, toutes et entières, ouvertes, sert dans la société masculine à alimenter un projet de société qui n'est pas le leur. Dans lequel elles ne se reconnaissent pas. Elles sont, au contraire, mises « en réserve de la nation ». Ce qui a pour effet de diminuer les femmes, de les menacer dans leur identité profonde.

Mais ce système actuel se trouve menacé lui aussi. Sa logique implacable, dichotomique, par son manque d'équilibre et de respect pour l'autre sexe, le conduit vers une catastrophe inéluctable (?). Il souffre de son obstination à nier son besoin et sa nécessité de l'autre sexe. Il a rompu un équilibre dans sa logique abstraite. Il est en train de détruire le sensible, le subjectif, le sujet.

L'apport du concept de plénitude demeure la seule approche véritable des femmes. Faire valoir leur différence, l'inscrire dans des projets particuliers obéissant à de nouvelles logiques; l'inscrire aussi dans les connaissances, voilà ce que peut constituer un potentiel révolutionnaire. La plénitude doit désormais constituer l'élément de base à tout projet féministe.

NOTES

1 « La préoccupation centrale des femmes pour l'art et la vie est à la fois le symptôme de leur marginalité professionnelle – d'une difficulté à se constituer une sphère d'intimité, par delà le territoire familial et au-deçà de l'espace des institutions ... et l'affirmation d'une volonté de fonder, sur cette articulation, la contribution spécifique des femmes à la culture: *la résistance passionnée à la dissociation des mondes* » (Bernier 1986, 160).

2 « ... c'est vers 'la vie' qu'affluait toute l'ardeur de ma jeunesse, cet état affectif sans objet qui, à l'instar des états amoureux, s'épanchait même dans des vers, » (Andreas Salomé 1977, 38).

3 « L'oeuvre de ma soeur, ce qui lui donne son intérêt unique, c'est que toute entière, elle est l'histoire de sa vie ... C'est une âme passionnée qui s'exprime. » Propos de Paul Claudel décrivant sa soeur (Cassar 1987, 438).

4 « L'horreur que tu as manifesté ultérieurement envers ce qui te remémorait ces mois de bonheur, m'a toujours déchirée. Pourquoi les as-tu

stigmatisés? Ils étaient l'expression de ce qu'il y avait de meilleur, de plus rayonnant, de plus fervent en nous » (Bourin 1980, 33). Ces sentiments traduiraient-ils également les sentiments de l'auteure Jeanne Bourin.

BIBLIOGRAPHIE

Andréas Salomé, L. 1977. *Ma vie.* Paris: PUF.

Bertrand, M., A. Casanova, *et al.* 1987. *JE. Sur l'individualité.* Paris: Éd. Sociales.

Bourin, J. 1980. *Trés sage Héloïse.* Paris: Éd. la Table Ronde.

Cassar, J. 1987. *Dossier Camille Claudel.* Paris: Éd. Seguiers.

de la Durantaye, C.V. 1988. « Essai sur l'épistémologie, les femmes et les valeurs organisationelles contemporaines. » Dans C. Baudoux et C.V. de la Durantaye, éds., *La femme de l'organisation.* Québec: PUQ.

French, M. 1980. *Les bons sentiments.* Paris: Éd. Acropole.

Harding, S. and N.B. Hintikka 1983. *Discovering Reality: Feminist Perspectives on Epistemology, Metaphysics, Methodology, and Philosophy of Science.* Boston: Dondretch.

Irigaray, L. 1984. *Éthique de la différence sexuelle.* Paris: Éd. de Minuit.

Irigaray, L. 1987. *Sexes et parentés.* Paris: Éd. de Minuit.

Jacob, F. 1981. *Le jeu des possibles.* Paris: Éd. Fayard.

Jacquard, A. 1982. Au péril de la science. Paris: Éd. du Seuil.

Kristeva, J. 1980. *Soleil noir: dépression et melancholie.* Paris: Gallimard.

Kuhn, T.S. 1983. *La structure des révolutions scientifiques.* Paris: Flammarion.

Lefebvre, H. 1969. *Logique formelle, logique dialectique.* Paris: Éd. Anthropos.

Lefebvre, H. 1985. *Qu'est-ce que penser?* Paris: Éd. Publisud.

Lindsay, C. and L. Duffin 1985. *Women and Work in Pre-industrial England.* Croom Helm: Oxford Women's Series.

Lyotard, J.F. 1979. *La condition post-moderne.* Paris: Éd. de Minuit.

Marcil-Lacoste, L. 1983. « The Trivialization of the Notion of Equality. » In S. Harding and N.B. Hintikka, eds., *Discovering Reality: Feminist Perspectives on Epistemology, Metaphysics, Methodology, and Philosophy of Science.* Boston: Dondretch.

Meister, A. 1975. *L'information créatrice.* Paris: PUF.

Norwood, R. 1986. *Ces femmes qui aiment trop.* Montréal: Stanké.

Perreault, I. et L. Bernier 1986. In I.Q.R.C. *Questions de culture* 9:160.

Thomas, L.V. 1979. *Civilisation et divigations.* Paris: Petite Bibliothèque Payot.

ELAYNE M. HARRIS

Well-Being for Rural Women: Empowerment through Nonformal Learning

Adults experience well-being when they learn and when their environment supports and encourages learning. Memorial University's Extension Service engages women who are involved in the community in their roles as mothers, wives, citizens, and volunteers, through nonformal learning activities which build capacity and self-esteem and contribute to well-being and empowerment. The opportunity for nonformal learning arises when women need new knowledge or skill to accomplish a particular task. Additionally, Extension staff help community women develop generic skills in problem solving and decision making. When the process is complete, women set their own learning agenda and use the community as a resource for their learning.

Le mieux-être des femmes en milieu rural:
l'acquisition de pouvoir par l'auto-apprentissage

Les adultes éprouvent un sentiment de bien-être en apprennant et quand leur milieu appuie et stimule cet apprentissage. Le Service d'éducation permanente de l'Université Memorial attire les femmes qui sont engagées dans leur communauté en tant que mères, épouses, citoyennes et bénévoles par le biais d'activités d'auto-apprentissage qui permettent d'acquérir des aptitudes qui mènent à un meilleur estime de soi, contribuant ainsi au mieux-être et à l'acquisition de pouvoir. Le besoin d'auto-apprentissage se fait sentir lorsque les femmes doivent acquérir de nouvelles connaissances ou aptitudes pour s'acquitter d'une tâche particulière. Le personnel du service aide en outre les femmes de la communauté à acquérir des aptitudes générales dans les domaines de la résolution des problèmes et de la prise de décisions. Une fois le processus terminé, les femmes établissent leur propre programme d'apprentissage et utilisent la communauté comme ressource pour leur apprentissage.

During the 1970s, a number of people in the allied fields of developmental psychology, educational gerontology, and thanatology reported that adults experience a sense of well-being when they learn and when their environment supports and encourages learning. That sense of well-being is attributable to an increase in, or maintenance of, self-esteem that can be associated with learning, if the environment is free from fear of failure or ridicule and when there is a positive attitude towards the capacity and ability to learn.

In Canada, as in other industrialized countries, every person must attend school for a period of ten to twelve years. With the exception of family, schooling is arguably the single most influential factor in the life of the child. The main role for a child between the ages of five (or six) and sixteen (to eighteen) is that of student. Schooling has within it well-established measures of success or failure – marks, regular progression through one grade per year, and eventually successful completion of all compulsory schooling; these measures and standards apply to everyone who participates. From this perspective, school is a common reference point used by both individuals and society at large to judge capacity, capability, and potential. In a society that increasingly values credentials, those who fail to graduate from high school are often perceived by others and themselves as failures.

In Newfoundland, we have some staggering statistics about early school leavers. For example, of those who began school in 1960 less than 40 per cent graduated. Less than 50 per cent of those who began school in 1970 graduated. Of these, about 45 per cent are women. On a more personal basis, of the women in my age group, less than half have had the positive reinforcement of successfully completing high school. I live, then, in a province where more than half the women of my own age have had an early serious challenge to a positive self concept and healthy self-esteem. Should anyone be so complacent as to believe that this is purely a Newfoundland phenomenon, a recent release from Southam News on Literacy in Canada estimates that 24 per cent of the adult Canadian population is illiterate. Newfoundland's illiteracy rate is admittedly the highest, but no one needs to minimize the effect of over 20 per cent of the female population of this country being illiterate. Since the Southam News report is based on the rate of literacy, not high school completion, the number of women in Canada whose self-esteem and well-being are seriously threatened simply through an experience they had before the age of eighteen, is higher than the 20 per cent who are illiterate. With this blow to self-esteem occurring at such an early age, many Canadian women have a considerable struggle to

reach a state of well-being unless they have cause to revise this formative perspective of themselves.

As an educator, I have noted that success in learning is a core
element in women's well-being. It is a challenge to find a means to
provide that element to many women whose past experiences with
schooling and the formal educational system were negative, debili-
tating, discouraging, and deflating. As an institution of higher learning, specifically university extension, our department is not by
definition one to which school leavers, illiterates, and drop-outs tend
to gravitate. In fact, we know that those who engage in traditional
university continuing education (generally consisting of courses,
seminars, and workshops) are usually those segments of the population which are already educated, employed, and in advantaged
socioeconomic classes. The university holds no threat to such
women; they are often its graduates. They have successfully navi-
gated their way through its institutionalized structures – registration,
course schedules, and examinations. It is therefore obvious that if
educators are to help women from other groups to have positive,
enhancing experiences that can lead to their well-being and empowerment, we need to engage them in learning that is nonthreatening,
not tainted with the structures or processes of schooling or formal
education that they associate with past failure, and free from barriers
of time, place, and fee.

A strategy that Memorial University's Extension Service has
adopted is to become engaged with women who are involved in
community activities in their roles as mothers, wives, citizens, and
volunteers. We try to help them realize what they want to do in these
roles in a way that involves nonformal learning and an enhancement
of their sense of capacity, self-esteem, well-being, and empowerment,
often without any of the women being initially conscious of the
learning process in which they have been engaged. In specific terms,
we place staff in rural communities throughout the province with
the task of helping community groups which are involved in activities
for community improvement. We do not offer courses or classes,
but we do engage women through committees, associations, or
special-interest groups in a process of problem solving and decision
making, or as we more commonly call it, community development.
The ultimate goal of community development as we practice it is to
help evolve a process of planning and action, a physical and social
environment that is best suited to the maximum growth and development of people as individuals and as productive members of their
society. Unlike others, who hold the view that community development (however worthy) is not compatible with the goals of an

institution of higher learning, we maintain with Haygood (1962) that
community development is essentially a direct method of teaching.
Instead of standing on the sidelines and assuming that instruction
done out of context (say, in a class) will lead to a productive attack
on local problems, community development helps the learner make
a direct connection between her learning and its application. We
may be dealing with concrete problems (the woman who is without
a job because the fish plant owner hires men first) or concepts (the
effect that make-work projects have on community life) but in any
case *relevance* is the chief characteristic of this approach.

Engaging women in nonformal learning through community development, for the benefit both of the community and the individual
herself, is allied with a view advanced by Alan Thomas (1978) that
much more learning is done in one's role as a member (of whatever
group) than in one's formal role as student. He contrasts the formal,
institutionalized, conventional role of student, defined and created
by organized education, with the role of member – behaviour that
is less formal, less conventional, and less associated with education.
The student role has characteristics of dependence, individualiza-
tion, self-consciousness, and market-orientation in that a service
(teaching) is bought. In contrast, the member has free choice of
participation when adults associate in a group of any size to achieve
a specific goal.

The learning element enters when the group as a whole or its
leadership realizes that, in order to accomplish the goal, some or all
of the group must acquire special skills or knowledge. Therefore,
learning is initially a means to an end and has acceptance and legitimacy because it is compatible with women's traditional and accepted role of concern for others rather than of self and self-
actualization. It is at this point that the role of the Extension development worker becomes paramount in creating the context in which
the desired learning or skill can be acquired and in which pride of
accomplishment and self-esteem can develope. For some women,
their learning as members of community groups is their first opportunity to replace their negative image of themselves as illiterates,
drop-outs, or school leavers, with the realization that they can, do,
and have learned.

The purposes of women's committees at the community level in
rural Newfoundland vary; such groups might include:

- Women who want to comment on topics of general concern in the
  community

- Women who want to focus on topics traditional to them in their
  roles as women – for example as mothers and wives

- Women who want to be fully appreciated for their contribution inside groups with both male and female membership

- Women who want to explore issues related to their status as women

Regardless of where women's groups are when they seek or encounter the services of Extension staff who can engage them in nonformal learning, there can be conscious efforts to foster self-confidence, organize group support and stress mutual self-help and assumption of responsibility for one's life. All efforts must be attuned to the overwhelming fear of failure and embarrassment that many women with negative schooling experiences must overcome before they can fulfill their learning potential. This kind of learning, which is cardinal to adult development, involves learning how we are caught in our own history and are reliving it. Women can learn to become critically aware of the cultural and psychological assumptions that have influenced the way they see themselves and their relationships and the way their lives are patterned. In women's groups which foster self-examination, women come to see themselves as having skills and abilities as strong as those who learn in the formal system and they use this realization to develop new personal and social action agendas. Through nonformal learning, they find a route to greater autonomy, control, responsibility, and empowerment. Whether they see themselves as having acquired the confidence to speak about a controversial community concern, or as joining with other women of the community in seeking a widows' allowance on the basis of the mining-related disease which caused their husbands' premature death, the community stage where women act out their various real life roles is where a great deal of important learning can take place. These possibilities are of vital interest to us as educators and feminists if we accept the premise that success in learning affects one's self-esteem and well-being and that after early failure with formal schooling, a significant proportion of women may be more willing to use the community as a place to learn than the more traditional setting of college, school board or university.

The challenge for community educators has a further dimension – specifically the task of helping women take the success of accomplishment in nonformal learning into a skill for their continued well-being. This involves helping women learn how to set individual learning goals and to locate the appropriate resources to achieve these goals – two critical steps in setting women on the path to independence and self-directed learning. It requires that the community worker help women understand how they can continue their learning without assistance from the Extension office. The individual herself can learn to take responsibility for the direction that is appropriate for her particular goals and interests, identifying her own needs, and recognizing the learning resources which are a part of her community and available to her. When these learning resourses are as varied as the person next door, a radio program, a skilled person in the neighbouring community, or the services of formal educational institutions, the learner will have a strong sense of her community. That sense of community can support and facilitate her individualized learning without undue reliance on any one source, and be an avenue to well-being that is available throughout a lifetime.

REFERENCES

Brundage, Donald and Dorothy MacKeracher 1980. *Adult Learning Principles and Their Application to Program Planning*. 2d ed. Toronto: Ontario Institute for Studies in Education.

Government of Newfoundland and Labrador 1986. *Education for Self Reliance*. Report of the Royal Commission on Employment and Unemployment.

Haygood, Kenneth 1962. *The University and Community Education*. Notes and Essays on Education for Adults, no. 36. Chicago: Centre for the Study of Liberal Education for Adults.

Leaving Early – A Study of Student Retention in Newfoundland and Labrador. 1984. St. John's. Joint Committee of Denominational Education Councils, Federation of School Boards, Memorial University of Newfoundland, Department of Education, Newfoundland Teachers' Association; chair: Dr. Thomas Pope.

Literacy in Canada. 1987. A research report prepared by the Creative Research Group for Southam News. Ottawa.

Mezirow, Jack 1978. "Perspective Transformation." *Adult Education* 28(2) 100–10.

Moore, G.A.B. and M.W. Waldron 1981. "Adults as Learners." In *Helping Adults Learn*. Guelph, Ontario: Office for Educational Practice, University of Guelph.

Thomas, Alan 1978. "The Adult Student: His Role as Student and Member." In R. Kidd and G. Selman, eds., *Coming of Age*. Toronto: Canadian Association for Adult Education.

Whale, Brock 1976. "The Community as a Place to Learn." In Harold Baker, ed., *The Teaching of Adults Series*. Saskatoon: Extension Division, University of Saskatchewan.

JOANNE PRINDIVILLE AND CATHRYN BOAK

Educating for Empowerment: Women's Studies as a Distance Education Course

Offering Women's Studies courses to off-campus women is a logical extension of feminist teaching and learning activities on campus. While universities provide a ready-made infrastructure for delivering distance education courses, they have developed their continuing studies programs for particular constituencies, using particular technologies. By examining the development and delivery of a specific multimedia distance education Women's Studies course, this paper addresses two issues: adapting university infrastructures and technologies to empower women off-campus, and coping with the incompatibilities between distance education delivery systems and the particular forms of teaching and learning to which Women's Studies is committed.

Éduquer pour permettre d'acquérir du pouvoir: études sur les femmes et télé-enseignement

Des cours d'études sur les femmes hors campus constitue le prolongement logique de l'enseignement féministe à l'université même. Alors que les universités possèdent l'infrastructure nécessaire au télé-enseignement, elles ont développé leurs programmes d'éducation permanente pour des clientèles particulières en utilisant des technologies particulières. En examinant le développement et la diffusion à distance d'un cours d'études sur les femmes à travers un système multimédiatique, cet article aborde les questions suivantes: comment utiliser les infrastructures et les technologies universitaires pour donner du pouvoir aux femmes hors campus; et comment traiter les incompatabilités entre ce type d'enseignement et les formes particulières de l'enseignement et de l'apprentissage propres aux études féministes.

CONTEXT

As we are often reminded by our colleagues, Women's Studies is an anomaly within the academic institution in terms of its theory and its practice. The academic legitimacy of Women's Studies is challenged both on the grounds that its definition of knowledge is unorthodox, including as it does the subjective experience of women and a commitment to social change, and on the grounds that the methods of teaching and learning adopted by feminist teachers are unprofessional or involve too much focus on applied work. The feminist assertion that "knowledge is power" disturbs academics who feel that only "unbiased" enquiry is acceptable. Our teaching methods may alienate administrators, whose jobs involve not only monitoring educational standards but also organizing the logistics of course delivery. In many ways, then, Women's Studies straddles the boundaries that academic institutions erect to create order by limiting and compartmentalising knowledge. These boundaries separate the pure from the applied, the objective from the subjective, the formal from the nonformal learning methods.

We argue that it is precisely in this lack of orthodoxy that the potential of Women's Studies for empowering women lies. However, insofar as we work towards this goal through existing educational institutions, we have to negotiate a workable compromise with those institutions, a compromise that allows us to benefit from the potential they offer while minimizing the obstacles they pose.

GOALS

Rather than developing knowledge purely for its own sake, the field of Women's Studies has an explicit commitment to the long-term goal of gender equality. None of us expects social change on this scale to be easily or quickly achieved. However, we do have a more immediate and more easily attainable goal: the empowerment of the individual women who take our courses. Various dimensions of Women's Studies contribute to the achievement of this goal. In an academic curriculum in which women are still largely invisible, Women's Studies contributes to women's knowledge of themselves and other women by communicating the results of feminist research. In place of theories and analytic constructs that ignore or trivialize women, their needs, accomplishments, and problems, Women's Studies offers feminist frameworks for both understanding and changing women's lives. In a society that isolates women from each other, Women's Studies makes visible the barriers that separate women and breaks these barriers down. In remote communities in which women struggle alone, isolated from feminist support systems and services, Women's Studies offers validation of women's perspectives. It affirms their struggles for equality and offers support.

AUDIENCE

One of the main objectives of distance education has been to reach out to female and male students who are beyond the unversity's walls. The possible audience for our Women's Studies course is very large – basically all the adult learners who can reach the university's teleconference sites in approximately fifty-five communities across Newfoundland and Labrador. Memorial, like many universities, has a mature student admissions policy for those twenty-one years old or older, so that a high school diploma is not a prerequisite for enrolment. If, however, over 40 per cent of the adult population of Newfoundland has ill-developed reading skills, as a recent Southam survey indicates, the potential audience for credit courses is greatly reduced, since the idea of a university credit course would be daunting or beyond the realm of possibility for thousands. Our Women's Studies course is a credit course.

Whom have we actually reached, then? The audience for the course has been relatively small and overwhelmingly female, ranging in age from nineteen to the mid-sixties, but tending to be in their thirties and forties. Students come from a variety of occupations and educational levels, from those who have never taken a university course to those with degrees. Their reasons for selecting the course also vary greatly: some students are actively involved in women's issues and take the course because they want to broaden their knowledge; others need a credit and can fit Women's Studies into their schedule and program. The following passages illustrate this range of motivations:

I work at a women's centre here in Labrador City and have been quite active in the women's movement for the last few years. I decided to try the Women's Studies course to see if I could get a bit more information on women's issues. [1]

I had a choice between this and physics. I didn't know if I could face a term of physics, so I picked Women's Studies. I hope it's going to interest me.

Some students identify themselves as feminists from the outset, whereas others are hoping to discover exactly what a feminist is.

Some are afraid they may not belong in the class because they don't think of themselves as feminists and believe Women's Studies is only for the converted.

The extent to which students in any class are geographically and socially isolated also varies greatly. Some live in very small remote communities, where transportation in and out is difficult for at least part of the year. Others live in urban centres which are very accessible. The degree of support services available varies with the size and relative isolation of each community. By the term "support services" we mean access to community library materials; to women's centres or women's networks, which provide contacts, support, and information; and to administrative personnel from Continuing Studies, who provide assistance and information and solve logistical problems. Another dimension of isolation which we will be dealing with later is students' relative isolation as course participants. This varies with the number of students at specific teleconference sites.

PROCESS

We have introduced the goals of Women's Studies and in a subsequent section will consider the content of the course. At this point we want to discuss the processes by which the content is shaped and through which it is taught. While there is a wealth of literature on both the goals and the curriculum of Women's Studies, there is much less written about the processes of teaching.

In a recent article, Renate Klein (1987, 187) notes the lack of "reflective writings on the theories and practices of the ws classroom dynamics." Following her review of themes that could guide feminist teaching, Klein points out that "if ws is to keep one of its initial promises – to be the educational arm of the Women's Liberation Movement – then the 'hows' of ws (its teaching practice) are as important as its 'what' (its curriculum)" (1987, 202).

Since we are discussing Women's Studies by distance education, let us briefly review the goals, content, and processes of distance education. Its goals are well established; generally they are described in terms of outreach. Distance education has no content *per se*, since the curriculum depends on the particular discipline. Process is the most important consideration in distance education. Its literature is a literature of process – that is, how to accomplish the established goals of outreach and those of the specific discipline through a particular structuring of the course content. Distance education goals are accomplished through media or technologies that have structures of their own, which differ in terms of teaching and learning characteristics. These characteristics include the following:

- Presentational characteristics

- Whether the technologies are ephemeral or permanent

- The structure/style of teaching material they allow: for example, how flexible they are

- Whether they permit interaction with learners

- The type of learning responses encouraged – surface or deep comprehension, analysis, problem solving, interpretation

- Distributional factors: whether the technologies work one-to-one, one-to many, or in networks (Bates 1987).

Distance education in Newfoundland has moved a long way from the days in which an itinerant teacher or a correspondence manual were the only choices available. The emphasis today is on using a combination of technologies in order to accentuate their strong points in relation to the goals of the course while minimizing their weaknesses. However, as Tony Bates of the British Open University notes, the selection and combination of technologies is complicated by the fact that their "appropriateness for learning tasks" comes last in determining what technologies are used in distance education. According to Bates, the relevant factors, in order of influence, are:

- Access

- Costs and numbers of students

- Organizational and political factors

- Teacher factors: time, training

- Student control, and

- Appropriateness for learning tasks (Bates 1987).

When you combine the lack of a definitive Women's Studies teaching dynamic with the many factors considered in techniques for distance education which come before their suitability for learning, the inescapable conclusion is that there is no one best way to shape a course. In considering the technologies used in our course, we will try to be candid about their selection and to look frankly at the opportunities and limitations they create.

Very briefly, the choices we made were print, video, film, and teleconferencing. Other possibilities include audio tape, computer-programmed feedback, and computer conferencing.

Print

At Memorial, print is the standard medium, except when it can be demonstrated that other technologies can do a better job. Most of us are so accustomed to working with print media, to reading print written by other people and creating our own, that we take it for granted. However, our distance education students do not necessarily handle print easily, although it is the medium with which students and instructors usually have the most experience. In the Women's Studies course, we used printed texts, a book of readings, a manual, and students' assignments and exams.

Considering Bates's characterization of the teaching and learning properties of technologies, we can note that print is permanent and can be approached in a flexible way; for example, a piece of writing does not have to be read straight through from start to finish. It works one-to-one and, except in the case of assignments and exams, does not permit interaction with learners. Print demands an active response on the part of students as readers or writers and can elicit a wide variety of learning responses from them. It is perhaps the most effective medium for communicating and facilitating comprehension of theories and concepts.

Let's look a bit more closely at one type of print material. Instructors at Memorial University often produce their own books of readings. In this way, it is possible to increase the relevance of materials for students by making them more attuned to local situations. However, the preparation of such collections involves considerable lead time for gathering and organizing articles, clearing copyright, and printing. The time and effort involved result in added costs. From the point of view of instructors and administrators, then, the production process usually decreases flexibility and dampens enthusiasm for updating materials.

Considering the factors determining the utilization of particular technologies, we can see that print may be more or less accessible, depending upon the complexity of the materials and the reading skill of the learner. In relation to other distance education technologies, print is relatively cheap, easily reproduced, and the easiest medium for most teachers to create.

Video and Film

Two other technologies of basic importance in the course are video and film. These are visual media, using the camera to record and preserve over time people and events; to establish particular viewpoints; to explore or establish relationships; to juxtapose events, images or opinions that may be widely separated by time and/or space; and to make them available to an audience also separated from them by time and space. In the process, video and film can call forth a variety of learning responses. The ability of these media to evoke affective responses is particulary impressive. Video is rapidly becoming more accessible to distance educators through lower capital costs and to learners through inexpensive videocassette recorders (vcrs). Whereas video and film, which we distribute on videotape, are often thought of as passive media and as mass media operating from one to many, the vcr makes one-to-one distribution and use possible. At the same time it increases flexibility for students using the medium and the control they have over it. Although home video decreases problems of access for many, it increases problems for those who cannot afford to purchase a vcr. Although it increases convenience and flexibility for many students by giving them access to course materials within their homes, it may also serve to increase students' isolation by eliminating the opportunity to meet in a central site for viewing and discussion.

Video and film are costly. While we produced our own video programs in the form of interviews, graphics, photographs, quotations, and so on, integrated into lectures, we also purchased the rights to duplicate and distribute films produced by a number of companies. In making such decisions, time and cost obviously are determining factors. A more important factor, though, is that purchase allows utilization of a much wider variety of films than could be produced by one organization – films that offer compelling glimpses of the diversity of women's lives.

Teleconferencing

Audio teleconferencing is utilized weekly in the course. In teleconference sessions one or more students gather in a centre around a table with a speaker and individual microphones. Ours is a two-way audio system, permitting a speaker in any centre to be heard by all other centres on the circuit. Teleconferencing is aural, interactive, real-time communication. It is ephemeral, although a recording made at the main teleconferencing centre is available to students upon request.

Students vary in the extent to which they find teleconferencing accessible. While some find it easy to communicate over the sytem, others are very inhibited. As we use it, teleconferencing allows for contact on-line across the circuit of sites and off-line among the participants in any one site. The first is a benefit that everyone in the course enjoys, while the second is experienced only by those in centres where there is more than one student. In the latter, students often conduct lively off-line discussions among themselves. Missing out on this rich source of student interaction is frustrating for the instructor and other students, who have access only to what the participants say on-line. Having a mix of groups and solitary individuals across the circuit contributes to a very different experience of the course for students at different sites. In the following exchange, a student solicited reassurance from her classmates:

"Has anybody completed the book of readings, because I'm way behind up here in St. Anthony?"
"Don't feel bad, my dear, we in Stephenville, I don't know if we've read more than two or three readings altogether."
"Well, I won't go jump off the wharf tonight, then."

Because other media are available for the presentation of information and development of concepts, instructors at Memorial are encouraged to use teleconferencing for questioning, elaborating, applying new knowledge to personal experience, and giving and receiving feedback.

Home or Site: Consequences for Women

With the use of increasing numbers of technologies in distance education, we have seen a first shift from education centred in people's homes, relying on the correspondence course, to sites that form the nuclei of designated geographic areas, where films and videotaped lectures are shown and teleconferences held, and, more recently, back to individuals' homes, with the use of home video and computer conferencing. We wonder whether the potential consequences for women students of these shifting styles of distance education are considered or understood. The recent swing of the pendulum back in the direction of home study is a case in point. Studies have shown that the home is not a safe place for many women, let alone a place conducive to study, and that many women do a double day of work and are expected to be on call whenever they are home. Research has shown that women who do not have paid employment often have low self-esteem and feel isolated in their homes. These women need the support and encouragement of others. With little economic power, many women cannot buy themselves vcrs or computers for home study. Even if these items are present in their homes, women often do not feel secure in claiming ownership of them for their own purposes.

Women's vulnerability in studying alone at home is increased when the subject is Women's Studies. At the very least, some women feel that, in the eyes of their families, they need a justification for taking Women's Studies. The political intention of Women's Studies and the sensitive nature of its curriculum can make viewing at home difficult or even dangerous. One of the women said, "My husband said, 'Don't you be watching that stuff at home.'"[2] Another student commented: "My husband will be some glad when this is over!" to which another woman replied: "I don't know if I'll have a husband by the time this is over."

The second time this course was offered, we changed the viewing of videotaped lectures from a site-based to a home-based activity. This change meant that students had to have access to a VCR. Comments have been generally favourable, the main benefit to students in our view being that they can work at their own pace and can repeat material they find difficult. We do not know how many women are not taking the course because they do not have a VCR, can't get quiet times for themselves on their own machine or someone else's, or would feel intimidated listening to the tapes with family members or friends. We would have even stronger reservations about some of the films going home unless it were by the individual women's informed choice. These films are often compelling accounts of women's experiences. Students typically have not confronted the issues they raise, such as violence against women, and, judging by what they say, they feel their partners and families may be less prepared than themselves to do so.

The message here is not that we should shy away from home-based study completely, but that we should make decisions with the potentially positive and negative consequences for the woman learner in mind.

CONTENT

Let us briefly consider two components of our course content that are essential to the effort to empower women. At the same time, we will indicate how we use the available variety of media and technologies to communicate these components.

A major focus of the course is women's experience. To help students in understanding their own experience, the course offers not only feminist frameworks but also concrete information about women in Canada generally and in Newfoundland and Labrador specifically. Students see films about women's experiences in other areas of Canada and are encouraged to draw both parallels and contrasts with their own experience. Consider this reaction:

We discussed the film [about lesbian mothers] for a few minutes afterward and I think the majority of us felt that the film was very enlightening. I know that my own views toward lesbianism were rather narrow-minded ... and I think it made me a little more broad-minded. These people have a right to make a choice, and it doesn't mean that they're not as good a parent as a person who is heterosexual.

There has, as yet, been very little research on women in Newfoundland and Labrador, but we have been able to compile a package of readings and videotapes documenting local women's past and present lives. The videotapes are particularly important because they provide a record of local women speaking about their lives and work, an aspect of women's knowledge that has been ephemeral. Through the medium of teleconferencing, students are able to share their experiences and discover both the commonality and the diversity of women's lives.

The second course component that is essential to the empowerment of women is the focus on formulating strategies for change. Through readings, films, and videotaped interviews, students learn how feminist theorists in Canada and elsewhere analyze particular issues and the strategies they advocate for dealing with them. Through writing assignments, students grapple with the problem of applying feminist theories to the understanding and transformation of their own lives. In the teleconference sessions, students have an opportunity to discuss strategies for changing their communities, their families, their work environments, and their lifestyles, as these comments illustrate:

"Is there any way of educating husbands?"
"Try leaving the dishes there till they pile right up to the ceiling."
"In my case, they'd be washed, because I've got a dishwasher, but in other cases I know of they'd be there till doomsday."
"Leave them there till doomsday and go buy paper plates!"

PRODUCT

What tangible results can we see from the delivery of our particular course to women in communities across Newfoundland and Labrador? Comments students make during teleconferences and in course evaluations, as well as their written work on assignments and exams, indicate that they have gained both knowledge about themselves and other women, and feminist perspectives on women's lives:

I was thinking. This has brought up a lot of things to me ... I think that women are doing two tremendous jobs. They're doing a fulltime job at home being a wife, a mother, a housewife, and they're working outside the home. I don't think there's a man alive who can stand up to it, to tell you the truth. I said that to my husband.

What really bothers me is that I always considered myself pretty well a feminist and it's not until I'd taken this course that I've considered the implications of what really goes on. It's pointed out a lot of new things to me.

The transmission by the course of knowledge and perspectives is not confined to the students themselves. Course materials and insights are shared with families, friends, colleagues, and critics:

That was one of the most interesting books that I've ever read. I read it so that I couldn't put it down. I went out in the kitchen with it; I went to the bathroom with it; I went to the bedroom with it. My mother came down for the weekend and I told her that it was a book that she has to read.

This dissemination process is a very important one. In a context in which the only access to information about feminism is through generally unsympathetic popular media, the course gives us an opportunity to define who we are and what we want and to reclaim the label:

I'm sure that the majority of women, if they understood the issues and knew what was happening, they would realize that they are in agreement with the women's movement.

As they gain insights into their situations as women, write about themselves, and discuss their ideas with other women, the students' confidence noticeably increases. The course reaffirms their sense of themselves as important and accomplished people.

Students acquire vocabulary, concepts, and communication skills that enable them to articulate their new understanding and to respond to anti-feminist rhetoric. As one woman explained:

I tend to get myself into the occasional argument about women's issues, and, being a feminist in a small community, any time women's issues are brought up you're usually in the middle of it, so I thought this might be a good opportunity to pick up a bit more ammunition.

Especially through the medium of teleconferencing, the course uses the university's resources to bring women who are doubly isolated into contact with each other. In the process, the students become familiar and comfortable with a technology that they can use for nonacademic purposes, since the university makes the teleconference system available to community groups, as well as to students.

OPPORTUNITIES AND LIMITATIONS

Teaching a distance education course is a different experience than teaching on campus, and so it should be. To try to replicate an on-campus course for off-campus use is to ignore both the opportunities and the limitations presented by distance education. To have any chance at a successful merger, Women's Studies and distance education must be able to form a partnership that respects the goals and processes of each. There have been many doubts expressed about the viability of such partnerships; in particular, there have been fears that Women's Studies and women students will receive short shrift. Obviously, we believe that Women's Studies and distance education can work together effectively. We have briefly discussed each of the technologies we used in the design of our distance education course and have touched upon the opportunities and limitations each presents. Just as there is no one ideal feminist teaching practice, there is no one perfect method for designing and delivering a long-distance Women's Studies course. Any choice we make will present opportunities in one area while it inevitably limits the achievement of our objectives in others. The reality of distance education is trade-offs. In making any decision it is necessary to juggle: (1) commitments to a particular content and style of teaching; (2) the range of available technologies; (3) the variable conditions under which our students live and study; and (4) the opportunities and constraints imposed by the administrative structure.

As we already have indicated, to date we have not reached large numbers of off-campus women with our Women's Studies credit course. Currently, we are involved in the time-consuming process of building a constituency. Especially in a province like Newfoundland, we recognize that university credit courses cannot have a direct impact on all women. As one of our students said:

How do you educate women to the point where they'll say, "This isn't the way things have to be, let's change it"? You have to reach more people than the people who are going to take a Women's Studies course through university. This is one way, but it's reaching a limited audience, and change is going to come pretty slow if this is the only way.

We recognize the need for a broad definition of education and a wide variety of initiatives directed toward empowering women, but, at the same time, we feel that university credit courses are an important component of our ongoing, multifaceted effort to empower women.

NOTES

1 Unless otherwise indicated, all quotations are from the audiotapes of the 1986 fall semester teleconferences. Minor editorial changes have been made to some quotations to facilitate their presentation in this format.
2 This quotation is from the 1987 winter semester teleconference audiotapes.

REFERENCES

Bates, A. 1987. "Technology and Learning: A Balancing Act." Presentation for the Canadian Association for Distance Education, national teleconference, 4 June 1987.
Klein, R.D. 1987. "The Dynamics of the Women's Studies Classroom: A Review Essay of the Teaching Practice of Women's Studies in Higher Education." *Women's Studies International Forum* 10(2): 187–206.

MAUREEN LEYLAND AND MAUREEN JESSOP ORTON

Challenging the Barriers to Social Change[1]

This paper presents the experience of a research and development project to reduce adolescent pregnancy in Ontario. Research findings from the project's second report (1986), document first, the effectiveness of preventive programs (school sexuality education and public health family planning clinics), and second, inequitable access to such programs. An alternative rationale is offered to counter the following barriers to development: sexist and class biases, "red herring" tactics of organized opposition, and confusion concerning the issues. Attention is drawn to problem reduction as a crucial objective for program evaluation, the principle of public access, and misconceptions in certain policy and program strategies.

Défier les obstacles au changement social

Cet article traite d'un projet de recherche et de développement visant à réduire le nombre de grossesses chez les adolescentes de l'Ontario. Les auteures résument les conclusions de la recherche tirées du deuxième rapport (1986), et documentent l'efficacité des programmes de prévention (programmes scolaires d'éducation sexuelle et cliniques publiques de planification familiale) ainsi que l'accessibilité non uniforme de ces programmes. Elles offrent une autre argumentation pour contrer les obstacles au développement, tels les préjugés sexistes et sociaux, les tactiques de "diversion" de l'opposition organisée et à la confusion entourant ces questions. Elles attirent l'attention sur la diminution du problème comme objectif déterminant de l'évaluation des programmes, le principe de l'accessibilité au public et les idées fausses qu'on retrouve dans certaines stratégies relevant des politiques et des programmes.

An ancient Greek exclaimed "All is change." We can never put our foot twice into the same river. Today, Ferron sings: "Ain't life a brook ... just when I'm feeling like a polished stone ... something changes." For women, the important question is: how can we influence the process to achieve the changes we want to see, beginning with equality for women and greater social equity between families to raise all above poverty?

This project[2] of research and development aims both to study and to intervene to reduce the incidence of adolescent pregnancy in Ontario. The project is distinctive in three ways: our perspective on the problem, our research methodology, and our commitment to promoting the development of preventive resources.

Pregnancy may be unwanted by a woman at any age due to anticipated consequences for her personal relationships, her health, and her socioeconomic circumstances. The unwanted pregnancy has consequences that may cost her community either financially or through limiting her potential contributions. Pregnancy before young people have the maturity to be good parents is particularly costly to everyone. In industrialized societies, adolescence is a time for education and the development of skills for employment. Adolescence thus affects two dimensions of relations: the personal maturity and the economic independence of the individual. In the majority of adolescent marriages, only the woman is an adolescent.[3] Consequently, precipitation (by unplanned pregnancy) of an adolescent woman into marriage or cohabitation with a young adult man is likely to ensure her economic dependency, lower status, and lack of power in the relationship and thus to reinforce sexual stereotypes.

The cause of adolescent pregnancy, in our view, is not moral deviance. Rather, we see individual behaviour as influenced by a number of environmental influences. Environment includes the behaviour of many other people interacting with and affecting the adolescent – parents, siblings, other relatives, friends, neighbours, school peers, dating partners, rock singers, movie actors, teachers, doctors, nurses, ministers, social workers, public health board members, board of education trustees, members of parliament.

Consequently we make two basic assumptions:

- Today, young people need their first twenty years for their own growth and development, before becoming parents

- It is the responsibility of adults to ensure that adolescents have a real choice to be sexually responsible and avoid pregnancy.

SUMMARY OF RESEARCH FINDINGS[4] '

1 Prevention succeeds at reducing both the number of teenaged pregnancies and the rate of abortion. Contrary to opposition claims, access to preventive programs has NOT increased the incidence of adolescent pregnancy. Access to abortion services has NOT increased sexual and contraceptive irresponsibility, and has NOT led to rising rates of adolescent pregnancy.

2 Preventive programs have been developed earlier and more extensively in localities of high socioeconomic status and under the one ministry with a special budget (Health). (Our measure of socioeconomic status includes the following factors: postsecondary education of men and women, women's participation in the labour force, and women's income. We assessed the socioeconomic status of fifty-four localities in Ontario.)

3 Localities experiencing the greatest decline in rates of adolescent pregnancy have *both* school sexuality education and public health clinics providing family planning services.

4 We found that adolescents in localities of lower socioeconomic status have lower life expectations and limited life opportunities, less access to preventive programs and, if pregnancy occurs, less access to abortion services. They are seriously disadvantaged simply by place of residence. The locality experiences a more rapid generational cycle of disadvantaged families.

CHALLENGES FOR CHANGE

To bring these research findings to the attention of concerned people, we have employed a range of strategies. These include three reports, two briefs to the Ontario government, endorsement of the briefs by thirty-three organizations to date, media conferences, many presentations to professional and community groups, and a brief to amend the proposed new Health Promotion and Protection Act. What have we learned in the course of these development activities? We have encountered a number of barriers, which we prefer to call challenges. These challenges are to be found in the process of change concerning any problem.

ATTITUDES AND BIASES

Even given intellectual awareness of a problem, frequently we are unaware of our own attitudes and biases that inhibit or divert us from acting to prevent the problem. Following are some illustrations of attitudes and biases that we encountered in some public officials and that obviously need to be reexamined in the light of current facts and evolving values.

Sexism

"These girls will just have to learn they can't trust those guys." When one of the authors of this report replied, "I really don't want to teach young girls they can *not* trust young men," he replied, "Well you can't, can you?" The underlying assumption here is that men are essentially sexually exploitative and incapable of being taught to be more trustworthy and responsible, and that young women must both bear the responsibility for protecting themselves from universally exploitive men and become the moral guardians for both. The implications of this biased assumption are obviously unacceptable – that is, that we should deliver sexuality education primarily or solely to young women. Unfortunately; the reality is that few young men enrol in *optional* courses on Health or Family Studies. Even in *required* physical and health education courses, male students are likely to have less class time for human sexuality than female students because they spend more time on competitive sports.

"What's wrong with adolescents having kids as long as they are married?" This bias confines its concern to the legitimation of children by marriage. It fails to recognize that young women need education and work skills just as much as young men. It assumes that a woman's life will be confined, largely or totally, to the private sphere – marriage and parenthood. It denies her need for and her right to an education and skills to enable her to make a contribution to the public sphere – through employment or public office.

Class Bias

"Half the world has been born to adolescent mothers; what's wrong with that?" This statement denies the need for social improvement in light of our extensive knowledge of the consequences of early and repeated pregnancies in women around the world: high maternal and infant mortality and morbidity. Nor does it take into consideration differences in the status of women around the world – real differences in ability to take more control over their lives. It does not recognize the changing roles of women and men in Western countries and the right of women to be well equipped to play their full part as self-sufficient human beings in all spheres of life.

"Those girls in the north end are just going to work in a factory or an office for a few years and then start their family ... so what does it matter if they get pregnant at eighteen rather than twenty-one?" This comment assumes that women in low-income neighbourhoods never have life expectations beyond an interim low-skilled and poorly paid job before establishing themselves as wives and mothers. In effect, this bias allows influential community members to define the life goals of low-income women. It denies them the right to choose their own life expectations and also denies the resources that would enable them to make sexual and reproductive decisions necessary to follow through on such life expectations. This denial limits life expectations for all members of low-income families. Classism and sexism combine in adolescent pregnancy to perpetuate the cycle of disadvantaged families.

Negative Assumptions Concerning Human Nature

"Kids don't have values." "You can't teach adolescents to make decisions; adolescence is an irrational stage in growing up." These comments assume that the capability and opportunity for decision making suddenly materialize at some entry point into adulthood. It denies the fact that learning is a continuous process from the moment of birth. Learning is applied to decision making through all life stages and life circumstances. Adults as well as adolescents can be irrational or rational in making decisions.

"Sex education is to striptease the mind." There is an assumption here that any information or discussion of sexuality is provocative and seductive and that it leads to sexual activity. Similarly, it is assumed that ignorance equals *a*sexuality, which we know to be absurd. Research demonstrates that, in the absence of sex education, misinformation and curiosity frequently lead to sexual activity.

"Contraception leads to promiscuity." "Contraception is an example of the lifeboat theory."[5] These statements assume that fear of pregnancy is the only deterrent to indiscriminate sexual intercourse, and that we have no other grounds for judgement in determining our sexual relationships. Surely this is an unacceptable assumption. Moreover, one of the objectives of sex eduction is to help us integrate values and morals into our decision making about sexual intimacy and contraception.

"If abortion services are available, then people won't bother to use contraception." This assumes that human beings are so irresponsible and self-destructive that they will plummet themselves into crisis

before taking action – that they prefer remedial rather than preventive action. We do not make this assumption when we promote
prevention of illness and disease or of accidents in the home, on the
road, and in the workplace. Why should we single out birth control
as the one area in which people are completely untrustworthy? Of
course, the application of the lifeboat theory to abortion services also
denies the real reasons for unwanted pregnancies, namely, lack of
preventive programs, inappropriate medical advice, lack of money
to buy contraceptives, uncooperative partners, or method failure.

These are just a few examples of attitudes and biases that we have
encountered. It is essential constantly to clarify our assumptions and
reveal any underlying bias.

ORGANIZED OPPOSITION

Misinformed Protest

Opposition to prevention does not always simply present a different
perspective on the problem. Following the release of the 1981 report,
opposition groups mounted a campaign which tried to discredit the
findings and block the development of preventive programs. One
group purported to present a critique of the report in its newsletter
but presented none of the findings. Its main theme seemed to be
that sex education and family planning did not prevent adolescent
pregnancy, but it provided no supportive evidence.

Shortly afterwards in the same community, 200 form letters were
presented to a public board of education by one of its separate school
trustees, opposing a proposal to develop a curriculum concerning
sexuality topics. Public agencies necessarily feel very vulnerable in
the face of such visible evidence of opposition, but they have no way
of knowing how well-informed the letter writers on the issue were.
In such circumstances, public agencies have a responsibility to ensure
that protesters hear an informed outline of the proposal, answer
questions, and clear up misinformation, rather than shelving the
proposal as too contentious.

Critical attention should be paid to "studies" offered by opposition
groups, studies which are often more opinion than research. The
handling of statistical data is frequently confused and erroneous.
They rely heavily on United States material, but the trends there
are different from Canada's. Moreover, lacking firm abortion statistics, United States researchers have not been able to demonstrate
the effectiveness of preventive programs as we have, using a broader
ecological framework and epidemiological method.

Discrediting Advocates of Change

The opposition also tries to discredit the agency advocating change. Its members may use the red herring technique; they try to divert the issue from sex education and contraception (that is, prevention) to abortion. In the context of pregnancy prevention, abortion is *not* the issue. The incidence of abortion may be an evaluative measure, since effective prevention of unwanted pregnancy reduces the need for abortion services.

We have been told that "Planned Parenthood is the greatest abortion referral agency in the country." Such a biased statement ignores the reality that, by Canadian law, physicians have been the ones to refer women to abortion services.[6] Moreover, Planned Parenthood has been the pioneer in promoting contraception in Canada for the past fifty years. In fact, it is precisely the organizations opposing abortion that frequently oppose or attempt to impede the development of sex education and contraception services. The organizations opposing the family planning section of the draft Ontario Health Promotion and Protection Act were Campaign Life, Renaissance, and Parents for Responsible Education and Family Health. Conversely, the organizations promoting the development of sex education and contraception (Planned Parenthood, women's groups, professional associations, nonfundamentalist Protestant churches, organized labour, and so on) are often very much concerned with developing equitable access to abortion services for women.

The red herring technique also diverts the issue to one of choice between "artificial" and "natural" methods of birth control or to individual moral decisions to refrain from sexual intercourse. This obscures the legitimacy of the issue as one of individuals having a real choice of an effective method of contraception.

CONFUSION CONCERNING THE ISSUES

Prevention as Distinct from Abortion

Planned Parenthood firmly supports the right of reproductive choice – that is, the right of individual women and men to avoid, plan, and space pregnancies. Sex education and contraception are seen as preventive services, and abortion is only one alternative to unwanted pregnancy.

People who oppose both prevention and abortion are in effect opposing the basic principle of self-determination in reproduction. This is not an issue of choice versus no choice. Rather, it is an issue of *whose* choice. Will the choice be made by the woman concerned, or by her partner, her parents, the power group making government policy, the local program gate-keeper, or male leaders of authoritarian religious groups?

Values as Distinct from Morals

Underlying the view among certain groups that adolescent pregnancy is simply a problem of individual morality is the belief that these groups have an edge on the "truth" about sexual responsibility to which we all should subscribe. This lack of tolerance stems partly from confusion between values and morals. Morality can be understood as a way of being and behaving according to certain values. We may share similar values but live differently. Although many promote the value of sexual responsibility, we differ in our views of masturbation, sexual intercourse, contraception, and so on. Opponents of abortion present their belief as a fundamental value – respect for life. Others share the same value, but apply it in the moral belief that respect for life includes respect for women and their self-determination in reproduction. Our developing knowledge of the wide range of life experiences (and especially women's life experiences) enables us to reexamine our values and morals, which evolve accordingly.

This confusion about values and morals and failure to recognize the role of developing knowledge is increased by the isolating effects of religous doctrine. At a public meeting, a representative of the local Roman Catholic diocese presented a framework of Roman Catholic values for Family Life courses in separate schools. It included two basic concepts: human sexuality concerns the whole person, and human sexuality is related to all aspects of a relationship. However, these same concepts are to be found throughout the professional literature on human sexuality and are also the base for public school sexuality education. This was an important opportunity to affirm some common theory and knowledge between the perspectives of separate and public school systems. Public debate also is often polarized by the incorrect assumption that public school sexuality education does not teach values simply because it does not teach the beliefs of one religious group. By clarifying our developing knowledge and our (frequently) common values, we are more likely to produce policies and programs which protect individuals from adolescent pregnancy and sexually transmitted diseases, and also to preserve everyone's right to self-determination in accordance with her or his moral beliefs.

Sex Education Is NOT *Eroticism, Is* NOT *Pornography*

For some people opposed to sex education, a picture of a nude body is pornographic. They fear that any knowledge of sexuality will be sexually stimulating and will necessarily lead young people to sexual behaviour. However, education in sexuality is not only learning important biological, psychological, and sociological knowledge, central to human experience, but also developing awareness of attitudes, clarifying values and morals, and learning and applying problem-solving skills to making decisions about relationships.

It is important to distinguish between eroticism and pornography. Eroticism includes sexual excitement, sexual desire, and sexual love. All three are different and none is inherently negative. Young people need to understand that clearly. If sexual excitement and sexual desire are labelled as negative, then when young people experience these feelings, they frequently rationalize their guilt by trying to convince themselves that this excitement means they are in love or the other person loves them. They trap themselves emotionally rather than recognizing that this excitement may be a physiological reaction to physical proximity or contact, or an emotional reaction of passing significance, or even a strong emotional reaction derived more from stress in some aspect of one's life than from a sense of closeness to the other person.

Sexual love is a sexual expression of love – the potential enrichment of human intimacy, bringing joy and greater meaning to chosen, treasured human relationships. Pornography, on the other hand, is concerned with power and the sexual exploitation of others, involving violence and debasement of others.

Education in human sexuality should encompass the developing sexual feelings, the many life situations and concerns experienced by young people. Throughout the school years, education should help young people to learn from their experiences and to clarify their values in order to make better choices in relationships, and to avoid potentially exploitative sexual encounters. Judging by curriculum outlines, some Family Life courses are limited to teaching basic relationship skills.

PROBLEM REDUCTION AS A MAJOR OBJECTIVE FOR SEXUALITY EDUCATION

The educational objectives of sex education are usually positive and general – for example, to develop more informed, careful, responsible decision making. Positive, general objectives are encouraging signposts. However, they do not indicate in themselves the most effective strategy, nor do they easily yield valid and reliable indicators for program evaluation. Focusing on problem prevention provides the opportunity for genuine program accountability.

When we concentrate only on positive program objectives, in effect we are allowing ourselves to mask the realities of problems. We fail to teach young people the sub-goals and strategies to deal with the pressures of daily life. When problem reduction is not specified as a program objective, then it is easy to deny that there is any problem at all.

While some provinces recognize the right of religious boards of education to teach their beliefs, all boards are being challenged to be accountable by evaluating their sexuality education with the criterion of reducing local adolescent pregnancy rates. Are these two objectives mutually exclusive? We think not. In our roles as educators and health and social science practitioners, we are beginning to subject religious beliefs and traditional values (which have not been evaluated in terms of preventing problems in this world) to professional principles of accountability. Furthermore, our concepts of equality and social justice demand that we review beliefs which result in the victimization of any particular group, in this case, women.

Among other objectives, sexuality and family life education should develop problem-solving and decision-making skills and promote the postponement of sexual intercourse until some appropriate level of personal development. The "appropriate level" is an important topic for discussion between parents and children and in educational groups under any auspices, precisely because the topic involves attention to individual developmental needs, life expectations, risks, responsibility to self and others, the character of the relationship, common values, and different moral views.

Traditionally, the appropriate time for sexual intercourse has been designated authoritatively as marriage. However, the demand for premarital chastity has always been used to deny the need for knowledge and has thus ensured ignorance, misinformation, guilt, and lack of communication on crucial sexual and reproductive issues. It has left us a legacy of sexual and social double standards for men and women, the sexual and reproductive exploitation of women, the stereotyped and restricted personal development of both men and women, a high incidence of adolescent pregnancy and adolescent marriage (frequently in that order), the lower socioeconomic status of women, and the perpetuation of families in poverty generation after generation. Premarital chastity may indeed be the choice for some individuals, but it hardly recommends itself as either an appropriate or an effective central concept for public education in a country which seriously aims to achieve greater social equality.

Principle of Public Access

In a democratic society, respect for moral differences and individual's rights to self-determination is ensured by *equitable* access to public programs of prevention.

Let us focus for a moment, on the issue of access under public boards of education. Some separate school trustees, anti-choice activists, and Protestant fundamentalist groups have opposed and blocked proposals for curriculum development concerning human sexuality. In one Ontario community, three different proposals were opposed by adherents of these groups. Other groups then requested the right to present their views to the board, and much support for the last proposal was expressed by professional community associations and agencies and parent groups, whereupon the proposal was finally passed.

This was a very contentious but important learning process for the community. Public school programs cannot be limited to what is acceptable to particular religious groups. Otherwise, the public school system cannot respect the diversity of a pluralistic society. In order to protect individual religious beliefs, it would perhaps be a reasonable compromise to allow students upon request to opt out of certain classes.

Claims by any religious group to speak for anyone but themselves or for other than their internal structure of authority must be challenged. For example, the Office of Family Life of the Archdiocese of Toronto and the Ontario Conference of Catholic Bishops presented a brief to the Ontario Standing Committee on Social Development in regard to the proposed Health Promotion and Protection Act (1982). They stated, "in raising our concerns we do so not only in the interest of the large and growing Catholic constituency which participates in the public school system, but also on behalf of other considerable groups with religious and accepted value systems."

We must challenge such assertions from highly centralized churches that furthermore exclude women from their ministry and policy-making group. Women cannot participate equally in the formation or interpretation of the moral view of such churches. Public institutions must resist the influence of nondemocratic organizations when these organizations try to restrict the principle of public access to preventive programs and, in so doing, undermine the civil rights of all.

PUBLIC STRUCTURES: TWO STEPS FORWARD AND ONE STEP BACK OR *VICE VERSA*

As new knowledge becomes available, we have to be careful that it is not used in inappropriate or distorted ways that limit the potential of prevention. Following are two examples.

A study of unmarried mothers in Nova Scotia revealed both a lack of educational programs to prevent unwanted pregnancy and a lack of support services both during pregnancy and following birth (Macdonnell 1981). The provincial Minister of Social Services responded by excluding unmarried mothers under the age of eighteen from Mother's Allowance. If the safety net (public assistance) is removed, then presumably young women will not get pregnant. This response implied that the cause of the problem is the individual woman, who is assumed to be in complete control of her life, learning, relationships with men, and access to family planning services, and to be able to afford effective contraceptive materials. This is another example of the lifeboat theory.

More recently, in Ontario, a public health unit used our research findings to focus on the local problem of adolescent pregnancy and to organize a community approach to the solution. The unit's recommendations were a partial and somewhat negative approach to prevention. They requested agencies to inform adolescents about family planning clinic services and actively to assist in referrals. However, they also stressed educating adolescent girls on the harsh realities of life on welfare assistance. They failed to emphasize the necessity to change life expectations and the opportunity structure, to promote the development of individual strengths and skills, and to promote mutually responsible relationships between young men and women. Implementation is thus skewed in a negative rather than positive direction by its emphasis on instilling fear of consequences. Moreover, the realities of life on welfare may disillusion middle-class girls, but will still offer some measure of independence to girls of low-income families. Although such skewed implementation may reduce the incidence of adolescent pregnancy, it relies primarily on changing only *women's* behaviour, and it will fall short of reaching the *most disadvantaged women*. Sexist and class biases continue unexamined and the social inequalities unchanged.

CONCLUSIONS

The barriers we have described are encountered everywhere – from individuals (from policy-makers to neighbours) as well as from organized opposing groups – and they interact with each other. They constitute a causal context in which we all live. These barriers contribute to the problem and they ensure its occurrence. We must continue to advocate for the development of education in human sexuality – to legitimate the very process of social development – as we try to raise public awareness of need. We must evaluate our preventive programs as we try to be accountable to our young people. We must ask ourselves if we are really addressing the problem and if we are reducing adolescent pregnancy rates in our own community.

We must advocate the principle of public access to sexuality education and contraceptive services. Parents and churches will teach their own morals and individuals will try to make their own decisions. Public institutions must educate young people about their rights and responsibilities.

NOTES

1 Two papers bearing a relationship to this one were published earlier. They are: "Learning to Be Long Distance Runners in the Marathon of Social Change" (Leyland and Orton 1986) and "Organizing for Action: Challenges for Change" in *It Takes Twenty Years to Grow: Reducing Teen Pregnancy in Your Community* (Planned Parenthood Ontario, 1988). Also available in French.

2 Ontario Adolescent Pregnancy Project (formerly the Planned Parenthood Ontario Adolescent Pregnancy Project). School of Social Work, McMaster University, Hamilton, Ontario.

3 Over the last three decades in Ontario, the ratio of adolescent women to adolescent men in marriages has been over 4:1 (Orton and Rosenblatt 1986).

4 Orton and Rosenblatt (1986).

5 The "lifeboat theory" is simply an assumption that people will be less responsible if they know they can avoid the consequences of their actions – that is, they will not care if the ship sinks, as long as there is a lifeboat for personal escape.

6 Physicians had to apply to hospital therapeutic abortion committees on behalf of women they recommended for abortion services until the 1987 decision of the Supreme Court of Canada which struck down the abortion law as unconstitutional.

REFERENCES

Leyland, Maureen, and Maureen Jessop Orton 1986. "Learning to Be Long Distance Runners in the Marathon of Social Change." Hamilton: Ontario Adolescent Pregnancy Project, School of Social Work, McMaster University.

Macdonnell, Susan 1981. *Vulnerable Mothers, Vulnerable Children.* Halifax: Nova Scotia Department of Social Services.

Orton, Maureen Jessop, and Ellen Rosenblatt 1986. "Adolescent Pregnancy in Ontario: Progress in Prevention." Hamilton: Ontario Adolescent Pregnancy Project, School of Social Work, McMaster University.

Orton, Maureen Jessop, and Ellen Rosenblatt 1981. "Adolescent Birth Planning Needs: Ontario in the Eighties." Hamilton: Ontario Adolescent Pregnancy Project, School of Social Work, McMaster University.

MARGUERITE ANDERSEN

L'amour et le bien-être

Comme réponse au problème des femmes, l'article suggère d'appeler les choses par leur nom, par exemple de dire études féministes et non pas études sur la femme, de libérer l'université de ses structures hiérarchiques, et finalement de faire preuve d'une plus grande vigilance vis-à-vis de l'amour. En littérature, l'amour est souvent vu comme un élément déséquilibrant, du moins en ce qui concerne la femme.

Love and Well-Being

As an answer to the problem of women's well-being this paper suggests the re-naming of Women's Studies as Feminist Studies; an academic system with less emphasis on hierarchy; and greater watchfulness with regard to love, a phenomenon which in literature is often depicted as a loss of mental and physical equilibrium.

Je suis censée vous parler du mieux-être des femmes et je suis censée en parler en tant que titulaire d'une des cinq chaires d'études sur les femmes au Canada. Permettez-moi quelques remarques préliminaires: Au lieu de cette expression maladroite « sur les femmes », je préférerais employer l'adjectif « féministes »; les études que nous faisons sont en effet des études féministes, ayant pour but l'avancement ou, si vous voulez, le mieux-être des femmes. Alors pourquoi ne pas employer le mot juste au lieu de se cacher dans des digressions diplomatiques? Il est temps que nous disions en toute franchise ce que nous pensons. Nous ne nous en porterons que mieux. Il me semble qu'en tant que titulaire de « chaire » j'ai le droit et même la responsabilité de faire des suggestions. Ma première suggestion serait que nous disions les choses telles qu'elles sont, que nous nommions le monde jusqu'à maintenant si mal/mâle nommé.

Être appelée à occuper un poste parce qu'on est féministe, quelle satisfaction! D'ordinaire le fait d'être féministe rend la vie à l'intérieur de l'université plutôt difficile. Les cinq chaires, créées par le Secrétariat d'État sur l'initiative de Margaret Fulton, certes ont leur bon côté en ce qu'elles reconnaissent l'importance du travail féministe, en affirment la crédibilité, donnent à leurs occupantes le temps de réfléchir et leur permettent de dire ce qu'elles pensent. Mais en même temps ces chaires soutiennent le système hiérarchique de l'institution masculine. Et je suis convaincue que nous ferions bien de changer ce système de façon radicale. Je discute parfois avec des collègues l'idée d'abolir les rangs, les échelons du professorat. Travailler dans ce but serait peut-être une façon de commencer à changer le système. C'est donc là ma deuxième suggestion. Et si je dis peut-être c'est parce que, en tant que titulaire de chaire, je me méfie de paraître investie d'une autorité spéciale. Ce que je vous livre aujourd'hui, ce ne sont que de simples réflexions de femme.

Et j'en viens à mon véritable sujet. Je voudrais vous parler d'amour. Sans vous parler de ma vie dont une bonne partie a été dédiée à ce sentiment, avec plus ou moins de succès. Non, je vous parlerai brièvement de l'amour et de ses effets sur la vie des femmes jeunes, tels que décrits dans les textes littéraires. Ceci constituera les fondements de ma troisième suggestion, qui serait que nous examinions, toujours dans le but de veiller au mieux-être des femmes, la question de l'amour et du mal-être qui semble, au moins en littérature, en résulter pour les femmes jeunes.

L'amour, me dit mon *Robert méthodique* de 1982, le premier *Robert* à avoir été préparé par une équipe essentiellement composée de femmes, « est une inclination envers une personne, le plus souvent à caractère passionnel, fondée sur l'instinct sexuel ». La passion, me dit-il et cela s'applique sans aucun doute à passionnel aussi, peut être « un état affectif prédominant », la passion peut être « subite, aveugle, aliénante ». Holà! « L'instinct », et cela vaut pour l'instinct sexuel, serait une « tendance innée à des actes déterminés, exécutés parfaitement sans expérience préalable ». Voilà des mots forts, des mots qui laissent entrevoir des dangers, des effets peut-être déséquilibrants. Je regarde sous « tomber amoureux », ça se trouve en voisinage direct avec tomber malade. « Tomber en amour » n'y figure pas, mais « tomber en » a toutes sortes de connotations négatives, comme « tomber en poussière, en ruines ».

Mais assez de fouiller le dictionnaire, allons donc nous regarder dans le miroir des vrais textes. D'après Michelle Coquillat (1982, 99), dans *La Poétique du mâle*, les xviie et xviiie siècles ont vu la dégradation de l'amour qui devient alors attaque subite, malheur, maladie, mort. « La dégradation de l'amour entraîne la dégradation de la femme sans laquelle il n'existe pas ... Face à l'homme qui a une essence divine ... la femme est définie comme la créature de la créature ... son milieu est l'arbitraire et la déraison ». Il est évident que la femme ne peut contribuer à la vie publique, ni à la création intellectuelle ou artistique.

Pourtant, le premier roman psychologique de la littérature française, *La Princesse de Clèves* (1678), est écrit par une femme, Mme de Lafayette. La Princesse de Clèves a appris de sa mère à se méfier de l'amour qui n'entraîne que du désordre. Elle se marie avec M. de Clèves parce qu'il faut bien se marier, tombe amoureuse de M. de Nemours et, après la mort de son mari qu'elle a tué en lui avouant sa faute, s'enferme dans la tranquillité d'un couvent pour échapper à cette passion nécessairement négative. D'après Coquillat, cette vision négative de l'amour et de la femme et, en parallèle, la survalorisation de l'homme, continue jusqu'en 1938, date de la publication de *La nausée* de Jean-Paul Sartre qui, en créant l'anti-mâle Roquentin, revalorise la femme et lui réattribue en même temps son pouvoir de création.

Au xviiie siècle, Rousseau avait confirmé la position inférieure de la femme, cause d'ennui et du mal, et insisté sur la nécessité de l'éduquer en vue de sa destinée de douce et patiente épouse et mère nourricière. L'amour, dans tout cela? Julie de Lespinasse affirme aimer « comme il faut aimer, dans le désespoir ». Au xixe siècle, Ellénore, dans *Adolphe* (1816) de Benjamin Constant, meurt d'amour. Dans *Madame Bovary* (1857), de Flaubert, l'amour mène Emma Bovary à la mort. Et malgré Sartre, tout cela ne prend pas fin en 1938. Dans *Les stances à Sophie*, Christiane Rochefort analyse en 1978 comment sa jeune protagoniste se perd, une fois amoureuse, comment en effet elle en devient malade. Marie Susini, dans *Un pas d'homme*, montre encore en 1974 une femme qui se croit incapable de fonctionner sans l'homme.

Marguerite Duras (1984, 39), dans ce magnifique roman d'amour qu'est *L'amant*, (1984) décrit ainsi la première rencontre de la jeune fille aux souliers dorés et au chapeau d'homme, couleur bois de rose: « Elle entre dans l'auto noire. La portière se referme. Une détresse à peine ressentie se produit tout à coup, une fatigue, la lumière sur le fleuve qui se ternit, mais à peine. Une surdité très légère aussi, un brouillard, partout. »

Et la jeune protagoniste, de concert avec l'écrivaine âgée, conclut: « Et je serai toujours là, à regretter tout ce que je fais, tout ce que je laisse, tout ce que je prends, le bon comme le mauvais » (40).

Elisabeth, dans *Kamouraska* par Anne Hébert (1970) est incomprise et par conséquent malheureuse. Thérèse, dans *Une forêt pour Zoé*, de

Louise Maheux-Forcier (1972) est incapable d'écrire le roman qu'elle voudrait entreprendre, tant elle est secouée par la passion. Marian, dans *La femme comestible* de Margaret Atwood (1969), est prise de vertige et de nausée devant l'idée du mariage.

Je ne suis pas sûre que Michelle Coquillat ait raison de dire que la dégradation de l'amour débute au xviie siècle et que c'est à partir de cette époque que l'amour, force négative, entraîne le mal-être de la femme. L'histoire est bien plus ancienne. Je vous cite Sappho: « Dès que je t'aperçois un instant, il ne m'est plus possible d'articuler une parole: ma langue se brise, sous ma peau, soudain, se glisse un feu subtil: mes yeux sont sans regard, mes oreilles bourdonnent, la sueur ruisselle de mon corps, un frisson me saisit toute; je deviens plus verte que l'herbe, et, peu s'en faut, je me sens mourir. » (Barthes 1977, 186).

Notons que les écrivaines que j'ai citées sont, soit d'une autre époque que la nôtre, soit, à l'exception d'Atwood et de Susini, au moins de ma génération ou même plus âgées. En général, elles voient l'amour comme cause de déséquilibre, de mal physique et mental. Atwood termine *La femme comestible* (1969), *Faire surface* (1972), et *La servante écarlate* (1986) en faisant allusion à une solution possible en la compagnie de l'homme. Est-ce parce qu'elle est plus jeune, plus optimiste, qu'elle affirme l'amour? Roland Barthes, un des hommes prêt à accepter ce qu'il y a en lui de féminin, écrit: « En dépit des difficultés de mon histoire, en dépit des malaises, des doutes, des désespoirs, en dépit des envies d'en sortir, je n'arrête pas d'affirmer en moi-même l'amour comme une valeur. » (1977, 29)

L'amour malaise, l'amour-valeur ... Le mieux-être des femmes auquel travaillent les féministes entraîne-t-il également un mieux-être en amour? Il faudrait, et c'est donc là ma troisième suggestion, aller vérifier dans les écrits des jeunes écrivaines si Simone de Beauvoir (1949, 415) avait raison en écrivant dans *Le deuxième sexe* que le changement de son statut en général permettra à la femme « d'aimer dans sa force, non dans sa faiblesse » et que grâce à ce changement, « l'amour deviendra pour elle comme pour l'homme source de vie et non de mortel danger ».

BIBLIOGRAPHIE

Barthes, Roland 1977. *Fragments d'un discours amoureux*. Paris: Seuil.
de Beauvoir, Simone 1949. *Le deuxième sexe*. Paris: Gallimard.
Coquillat, Michaelle 1982. *La Poétique du mâle*. Paris: Gallimard.
Duras, Marguerite 1984. *L'Amant*. Paris: Éditions de Minuit.

Contributors
Collaboratrices

MARGUERITE ANDERSEN, professeure et écrivaine, a été titulaire de la chaire d'études féministes à l'Université Mont Saint-Vincent de 1987 à 1988. Auteure d'études critiques, d'un roman (1982), de nouvelles et d'un recueil de poèmes en prose (1984), elle a été l'éditrice de *Mother was not a person* (1972), titre classique du féminisme canadien. La traduction en anglais de son recueil de poèmes en prose, *L'Autrement pareille* – qui traite de la relation mère-fille – paraîtra en 1990.

CAROLINE ANDREW est professeure au départment de science politique de l'Université d'Ottawa. Elle mène en collaboration avec Cécile Coderre et Ann Dennis un projet de recherche sur les femmes cadres.

MONIQUE BÉGIN PC, completed a master's degree in sociology at the University of Montréal and doctoral studies at the Sorbonne in Paris. From 1967 to 1970, she served as the Executive Secretary of the Royal Commission on the Status of Women in Canada, and co-signed the report to Parliament. She was elected to the House of Commons in October 1972 as the first woman MP from Quebec and was re-elected in 1974, 1979, and 1980. She served as minister of National Health and Welfare from 1977 to 1984. She has been a university professor since 1984. Currently she is joint chair in Women's Studies at the University of Ottawa and at Carleton University.

LESLIE BELLA has taught in Recreation and Leisure Studies at University of Alberta and at the Faculty of Social Work at University of Regina where she served as Dean. She is now a professor in the School of Social Work at Memorial University, Newfoundland, where she teaches everything from Women and Welfare to Communication Skills. Her degrees include an MSW from University of British Columbia and a PHD in Political Science from the University of Alberta.

CATHRYN BOAK is the Production Manager of the Telemedicine and Educational Technology Resources Agency, Memorial University of Newfoundland, which provides consulting, design, and production services in distance education and training. Her research interests include the analysis of teleconferencing as an interactive educational medium, and the implications of changes in families and the roles of women in Canada for educational policy and practice.

CÉCILE CODERRE est professeure au département de sociologie de l'Université d'Ottawa. Elle participe activement au programme des études des femmes et mène en collaboration avec Caroline Andrew et Ann Dennis un projet de recherche sur les femmes cadres.

DAWN CURRIE completed her undergraduate and graduate degrees at the University of Saskatchewan, and received a PHD from the London School of Economics in 1988. Her doctoral research concerned reproductive decision making and the deferral of childbearing. Dawn's current areas of interest are feminist theory, women and law/justice, and aspects of women and medicine. Dawn taught Women's Studies for three years at the University of Saskatchewan but is now teaching in the Anthropology and Sociology Department at the University of British Columbia.

MEGAN BARKER DAVIES is an active feminist and a women's historian who is currently completing her MA thesis on the history of mental health patients in British Columbia. She has worked in the field of community mental health in Canada and Wales and has taught ESL in the People's Republic of China.

ANN DENIS est professeure au département de sociologie de l'Université d'Ottawa. Elle mène en collaboration avec Cécile Coderre et Caroline Andrew un projet de recherche sur les femmes cadres.

CLAIRE V. DE LA DURANTAYE est économiste. Après avoir obtenu un baccalauréat et une maîtrise en Science économique à l'Université d'Ottawa, elle obtient un doctorat de 3ᵉ cycle en analyse de politiques de l'École des Hautes Études en sciences sociales de Paris (1983). Elle enseigne actuellement au département d'administration et d'économique de l'Université du Québec à Trois-Rivières et poursuit une recherche, à titre de co-responsable, portant sur les obstacles à la promotion des femmes dans la gestion de l'éducation au Québec. Elle a également été vice-doyenne de la Faculté des Sciences sociales et de l'Administration à l'Université du Québec à Trois-Rivières de 1983 à 1986.

GLORIA R. GELLER is a member of the Faculty of Social Work, University of Regina. She completed her doctorate at the Ontario Institute for Studies in Education. She has conducted research on the differential treatment of males and females in the juvenile justice system. She is presently carrying out research on justice for women victims of abuse.

MADELINE JEAN GRAVELINE is currently an assistant professor at the Department of Social Work at St Thomas University in Fredericton. She has lived most of her life in rural and northern Canada and has been a very active participant in developing feminist groups in communities where she has lived.

NANCY GUBERMAN is a professor of social work at the University of Quebec in Montreal, where she teaches women's studies and community organization. Her research interests include feminist intervention, violence against women, and state-family relations as typified by family policy legislation. She is currently working on a study of the factors that lead women to take on the care of dependent adults in the family, funded by Health and Welfare Canada.

ELAYNE M. HARRIS has been the Director of Extension Service, Memorial University of Newfoundland for six years. She is currently on leave as a doctoral student at the Ontario Institute for Studies in Education. She has been active in national associations such as Canadian Association for Adult Education, The Canadian Association for University Continuing Education, and the Canadian Congress on Learning Opportunities for Women.

CAROL D.H. HARVEY is currently associate professor and head of Family Studies, Faculty of Human Ecology, University of Manitoba, Winnipeg. She was raised on a farm in Idaho and earned a bachelor's degree in home economics extension at the University of Idaho and later a master's degree in family studies and a doctorate in sociology from Washington State University. Her research interests are in widowhood and intergenerational relationships.

ANDREA LEBOWITZ is a senior lecturer in the Department of English at Simon Fraser University. Also a founding member of the Women's Studies Program, she is presently its graduate chairperson. Her fields of interest are the nineteenth-century British novel and feminist literary criticism.

MAUREEN LEYLAND is a co-director of the Ontario Adolescent Pregnancy Project and a past president of Planned Parenthood Ontario. She is currently in a study of equal pay for work of equal value, conducted jointly by the federal government and associated unions. She is a national officer with the Public Service Alliance of Canada (Canadian Employment and Immigration Union) with special responsibility for women's issues.

DORIS MCILROY, BA (Honours in Anthropology), MA (Canadian Studies) is a freelance writer and researcher, potter, and sports enthusiast.

KABAHENDA NYAKABWA earned a master's degree at the Department of Family Studies, Faculty of Human Ecology, University of Manitoba at Winnipeg. Her research interests are in refugees and immigrant family adaptation. She is a recent immigrant to Canada and a doctoral student in Sociology at Carleton University.

MARY O'BRIEN teaches in the Gerontology Department at Mount St. Vincent University in Halifax. Her research interests are in older women, particularly in the factors that enhance their ability to handle the changes which accompany the aging process. She has recently begun research on older women and spirituality.

MAUREEN JESSOP ORTON has degrees in social work and a master's degree in social welfare policy and is a doctoral candidate at the Faculty of Social Work, University of Toronto. She is a co-director and co-researcher for the Ontario Adolescent Pregnancy Project at the School of Social Work, McMaster University where she taught a course on human sexuality for six years. She is a founding member and past chairperson, Sexuality Committee, Ontario Association of Professional Social Workers.

JOANNE PRINDIVILLE has taught anthropology and women's studies at various universities as well as working as a consultant on women's issues. Her current projects include organizing community action workshops for women in Newfoundland and Labrador and working on issues concerning women in development in Indonesia.

MONIQUE RAIMBAULT was employed as researcher for the Consulting Committee on the Status of Women with Disabilities for two years. She has undertaken two research projects dealing with the realities faced by women with disabilities. Presently working for the Manitoba Action Committee on the Status of Women, she is involved in community organizing and political activism.

GHYSLAINE SAVARIA collabore depuis plus de 30 ans, à titre d'administratrice, à l'exploitation d'une entreprise familiale. Elle a participé à la fondation de l'Association des femmes collaboratrices, dont elle a été vice-présidente. Détentrice d'un certificat en relations publiques et d'un diplôme d'enseignement supérieur, elle est aussi formatrice à l'éducation des adultes, section gestion-économie.

EVA A. SZEKELY is a member of the Women Working with Immigrant Women in Toronto. She teaches women's studies courses part-time at the Ontario Institute for Studies in Education and works as a psychologist-consultant at Youthdale Treatment Centres in Toronto.